COLOUR GUIDE

PICTURE TESTS

Gynaecology and Obstetrics

Janice Rymer MD MRCOG FRNZCOG
Consultant Obstetrician and Gynaecologist,
Guy's Hospital, London

Enzo Lombardi FRACOG
Consultant Obstetrician and Gynaecologist,
Flinders Medical Centre; Lecturer in Reproductive Medicine,
Flinders University of South Australia, Adelaide

Churchill Livingstone

EDINBURGH LONDON MADRID MELBOURNE NEW YORK TOKYO 1994

Acknowledgements

Many friends, colleagues, relatives and patients have contributed to this book and we are extremely grateful. We would especially like to thank N. Baig, J. Higham, L. Holmesby, P. Knott and G. Mulcahy for generously giving their time both in photographing the patients and donating these slides. The following people have also donated their slides and we are very grateful:

W. McCullough	J. Slavotinek	C. Nelson
A. Rodin	G. Desia	J. Moir
A. George	P. Bobrow	P. Wilson
T. Coltart	S. Barton	T. Blackmore
D. Maxwell	C. Watson	C. Cooper
M. Chapman	Sir J. Dewhurst	S. Cooper
T. Clark	J. Parker	G. Hart
R. Forman	M. Stewart	R. Ing
A. Phillips	H. Issler	S. James
N. Holmes	P. Greenhouse	W. Jones
I. Tucker	R. Jelly	R. Leeson
L. Fisher	N. Beechey-Newman	S. Lombardi
I. Fogelman	H. Archibald	M. Penniment
A. Fish	F. Hook	R. Royal
I. Boyle	J. Treasure	S. Hussain
D. Steel	A. Sinclair	L. Burchell
S. Adeaga		

FMC Labour Ward Staff, Adelaide
QVH Ultrasound Dept, Adelaide

We would also like to acknowledge the Guy's Hospital Photographic Department which has cheerfully met ALL of our demands. The book would not have been possible without the Guy's Hospital Obstetric and Gynaecology Unit as well as the Department of Obstetrics and Gynaecology at Flinders Medical Centre in South Australia. We were amazed at the patients' willingness to allow themselves to be photographed.

We are most indebted to Julie White, secretary to the Department of Obstetrics and Gynaecology at Guy's Hospital, and Robyn White, secretary to the Department of Obstetrics and Gynaecology at Flinders Medical Centre. They have typed the manuscript and tolerated the endless changes with great cheerfulness and good humour.

1994

J. R.
E. L.

Contents

Gynaecology—questions   1
Obstetrics—questions   55
Answers—gynaecology   109
Answers—obstetrics   131

Index   155

Gynaecology—Questions

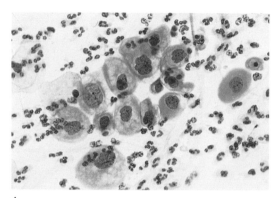

1. This slide shows dyskaryosis.

a. What type of cells are these?
b. These cells display some of the features of malignancy. Name them.

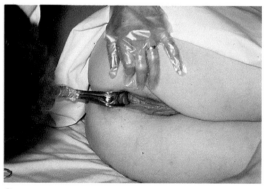

2.

a. What speculum is being used for this examination?
b. Describe the Sims' position.
c. In what circumstances would you use this speculum?
d. What other instruments should you use with this speculum?

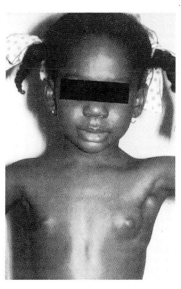

3.

a. What sign does this 6 year old exhibit?
b. What is the diagnosis?
c. What is the cause of this condition?
d. What is the treatment?
e. What is the usual sequence of development of secondary sexual characteristics?

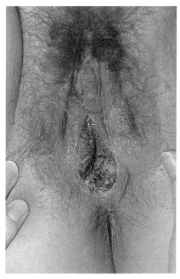

4. This young woman has undergone laser treatment to the vulva.

a. What is the most likely indication for this treatment?
b. What essential investigation is required before embarking on this treatment?
c. What are the potential postoperative complications?
d. What other treatment options are available?
e. How would you manage this patient postoperatively?

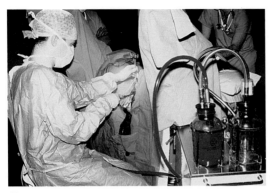

5. This woman is undergoing an early termination of pregnancy.

a. What are the legal indications?
b. What methods are available for termination of an early pregnancy?
c. What are the immediate and short-term complications of this procedure?
d. What are the possible adverse longterm sequelae?

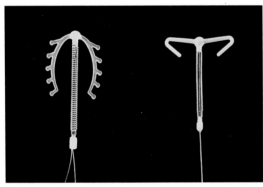

6.

a. What are these?
b. What is the mechanism of action?
c. What are the absolute contraindications?
d. Describe the mechanism of insertion.
e. What are the complications associated with their use?
f. How often should copper-containing devices be changed?

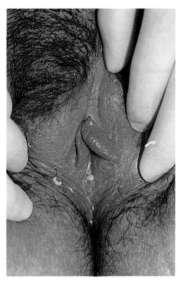

7.

a. What is the diagnosis?
b. What symptoms may the patient complain of?
c. How would you confirm the diagnosis?
d. What is the treatment?
e. How would you treat the recalcitrant case?

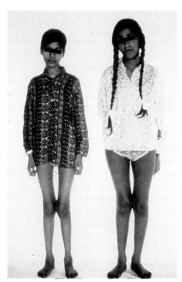

8. These girls have a bone disorder.

a. What is the diagnosis?
b. What is the pathology?
c. Do you anticipate any problems with childbearing?

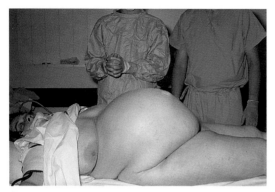

9. **This woman has a large mass arising from the pelvis.**

a. What are the possible gynaecological causes of the mass?
b. What are the more common nongynaecological possibilities?
c. What would be your diagnostic approach to this woman?

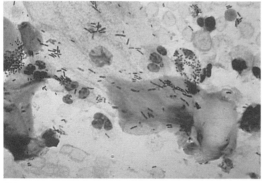

10.

a. What organisms are present on this Gram-stain smear?
b. What is the resultant clinical condition?
c. What are the clinical manifestations in females?
d. How is the definitive diagnosis made?
e. What are the principles of management?

INSTRUCTIONS		TOWEL	1	2	3	4	5	6	7	8
Name......	1p 2p		❮❮				|||	||		
Date period started					|||||	||	|||||			
1. Enter your name and the start date (first day of your period. 2. *Before you dispose of each towel or tampon,* compare it with the pictures on the chart. 3. To record the amount of blood loss, make a mark (I) in the box opposite the picture which looks like your towel/tampon. Make a mark every time you discard a pad or tampon — on every day of your period. 4. When you reach four marks (IIII), make the next mark like this (IIII). 5. If you notice any blood clots on the towel/tampon, or pass one in the toilet, write in the size and number each day. Guess the size by comparing the clots to coins (see exercises).	50p 6. If you experience any flooding, write F on the day it happens. 7. *Please do not forget* to return your completed chart(s) to the hospital/clinic. If you do not understand how to complete these charts, *please* do not be embarrassed to ask your doctor — it is important to complete the chart correctly.				|||	||||	|||				
		CLOTS		10p×2	50p					
		FLOODING	F	F						
	© Boobing/Wintbrop 1990									

11.

a. What is the purpose of this chart?
b. What is the normal menstrual blood loss?
c. What does this chart reveal?
d. What are the usual causes of excessive menstrual blood loss?
e. How would you investigate and treat this patient?

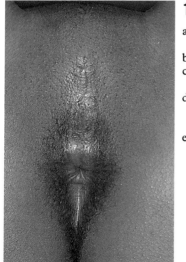

12.

a. What procedure has this young girl undergone?
b. How may these patients present?
c. What problems can occur in labour?
d. What elective gynaecological procedure can alleviate the problem?
e. If diagnosed in labour how may delivery be facilitated?

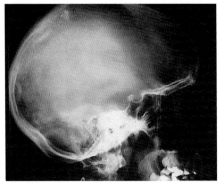

13.

a. What does this X-ray reveal?
b. What is the most likely cause and how would this patient present to the Gynaecology Department?
c. What other investigations would you perform?
d. Name other causes of hyperprolactinaemia.
e. What are the treatment options?

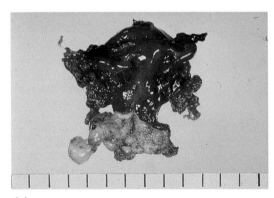

14. This specimen is a sarcoma botryoides.

a. What organ is affected?
b. What is the pathology?
c. In what age group does this lesion typically occur?
d. What is found on examination?
e. What is the pattern of spread?
f. What is the treatment?

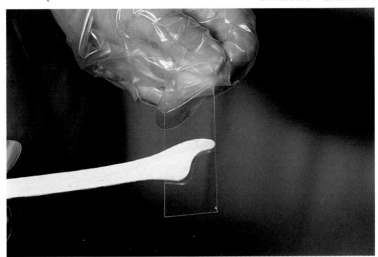

15.

a. What test is being performed and what is the purpose?
b. What is the name of the instrument?
c. How frequently should this investigation be performed?
d. What area must be sampled?
e. How can one optimize the sample obtained?

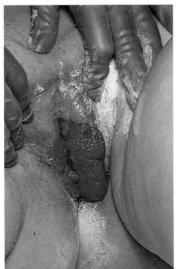

16.

a. What is the obvious diagnosis?
b. In what age group does this condition typically occur?
c. What is the usual histology?
d. What is the primary route of spread?
e. What are the principles of treatment?

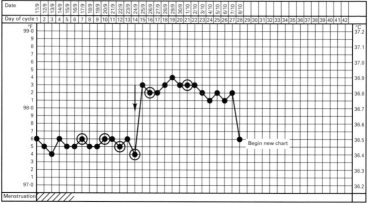

Month and year September 1984   ⦿ = Intercourse   ↓ = Ovulation

17.

a. What is the name of this record?
b. What does this record illustrate?
c. What event has presumptively occurred?
d. By what method can this event be more definitively diagnosed?

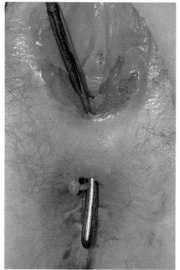

18.

a. What abnormality is being demonstrated?
b. What is the most common cause of a rectovaginal fistula?
c. What are some other causes of rectovaginal fistulae?

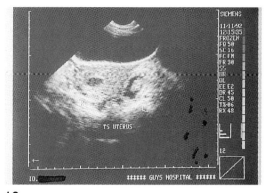

19. The photographs in questions 19–21 relate to a woman who presented with an unruptured ectopic pregnancy.

a. Describe the sonographic findings.
b. What are the classic symptoms of this condition?
c. What are the typical signs?
d. What ancillary investigations can help to make the diagnosis?

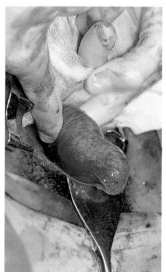

20.

a. What aetiological factors contribute to the incidence of ectopic pregnancy?
b. What are the common anatomical sites?
c. What is the natural history of ectopic pregnancy?
d. What is the differential diagnosis?

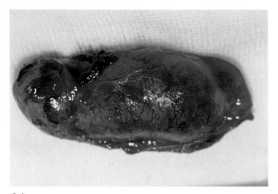

21. This patient underwent salpingectomy.

a. What treatment options are available in the treatment of ectopic pregnancies?
b. How would you counsel this patient postoperatively?
c. What is the recurrence risk?

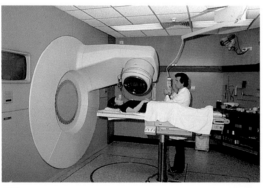

22. This young woman is undergoing radiation therapy.

a. For which gynaecological cancers does radiation therapy have an established curative role?
b. In what ways may radiation therapy be delivered?
c. What acute adverse reactions are seen?
d. What are the possible longterm sequelae of radiation therapy?

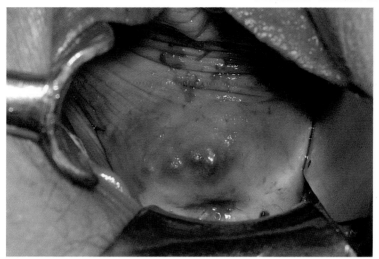

23.

a. What is the most likely diagnosis? Define this condition.
b. What are the theories of aetiology?
c. What are the symptoms and signs?
d. How could the diagnosis be confirmed in this case?
e. How is the diagnosis usually made?

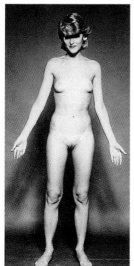

24.

a. Describe what you see.
b. What is the diagnosis?
c. What is the basis of this condition?
d. When do these patients normally present?
e. What else might you find on clinical examination?

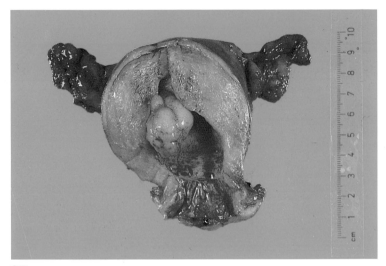

25.

a. Describe what you see.
b. What symptoms may these cause?
c. How may these be detected?
d. What is the treatment?

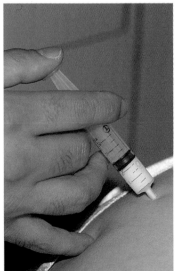

26. This woman is receiving depot medroxy progesterone acetate.

a. How does it work?
b. Is a steady dose provided?
c. What is the failure rate of this method?
d. What are the advantages of this method?
e. What are the disadvantages?

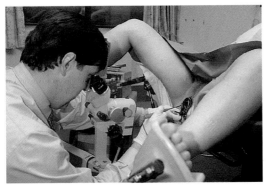

27.

a. What investigation is this woman undergoing?
b. Who would you refer for this investigation?
c. What basic steps are involved in this procedure?
d. How would you counsel a woman prior to referral?

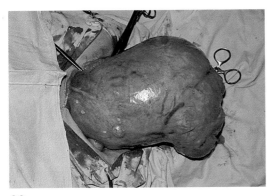

28. This is an intraoperative specimen of a woman who had iron deficiency anaemia.

a. What may have caused this anaemia?
b. What symptoms may she have presented with?
c. What preoperative medication can be prescribed to simplify surgery?

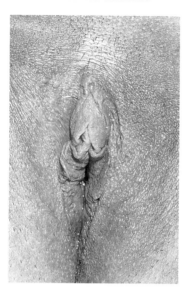

29. The photographs in questions 29 and 30 relate to a patient with virilism.

a. What sign of virilism is present?
b. What are other signs of virilism?
c. What are the causes of female virilization?
d. What are the sites of testosterone production in normal women?

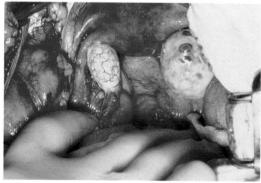

30.

a. Outline the diagnostic approach in a patient who exhibits virilism.
b. What cause of virilism is present in this patient?
c. Which ovarian tumours produce androgens and virilizing syndromes?
d. Which signs of virilism disappear after removal of such tumours?

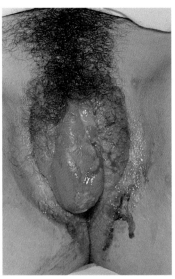

31.

a. What is the diagnosis?
b. What are the typical clinical features?
c. How should this condition be managed?
d. What are the obstetric implications of this condition?

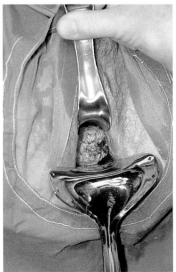

32.

a. What is the diagnosis?
b. What is the age distribution of this condition?
c. What is the typical presentation?
d. What is the characteristic pattern of spread?
e. How is this condition staged?
f. Define the four stages.

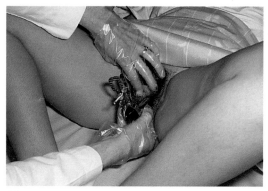

33.

a. What is this speculum called?
b. What position is the patient in?
c. How would you insert this speculum?
d. What examination would you use as an adjunct to the use of this speculum?

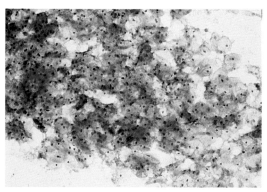

34. This is a vaginal cytology slide.

a. What hormonal pattern does this show?
b. What cells predominate?
c. Would the karyopyknotic index be high or low?
d. In what situations would this pattern be seen?

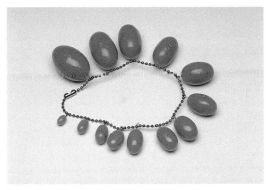

35.

a. What is this device?
b. What is the function of this device?
c. Describe the characteristics of a normal testicle.
d. What are the average dimensions and volume of a normal testis?
e. What are some causes of testicular atrophy?

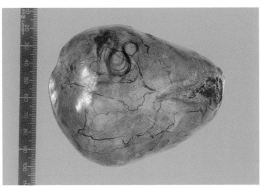

36.

a. What is the diagnosis?
b. At what ages is this typically seen?
c. What is the origin of the cyst? What tissues can be within it?
d. What is the incidence of bilateral lesions and what is the significance of this figure?
e. What is the malignant potential?

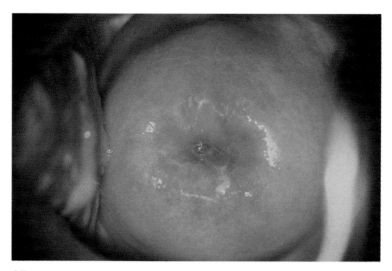

37.

a. What instrument is being used here and what does it show?
b. During this investigation what solutions are applied?
c. What is dyskaryosis?
d. What is dysplasia?

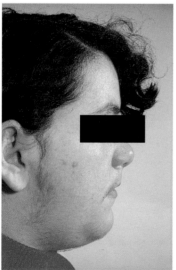

38.

a. What is the name of this condition?
b. What scoring system can help estimate the severity of the problem?
c. What are the common causes?
d. How would you investigate this patient?
e. What treatment modalities are available?

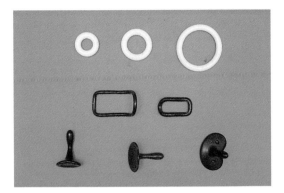

39.

a. What are these devices called?
b. Name the three types illustrated.
c. What are the indications for their use?
d. What potential complications can occur with their use?
e. How often should the white devices be changed?

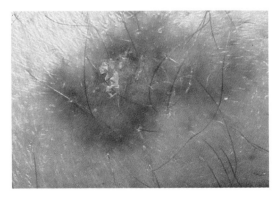

40. This slide illustrates Karposi's sarcoma in a young patient.

a. With what immunodeficiency state is this condition commonly associated?
b. Which individuals are at risk?
c. Into which fluids can the offending virus be shed?
d. How can the underlying diagnosis be definitively made?

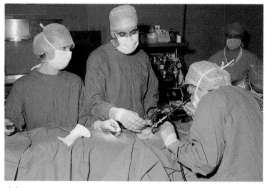

41.

a. What procedure is being performed?
b. What is the peritoneal cavity inflated with?
c. What organs can be visualized by this method?
d. What must be done before the Verres needle is introduced?

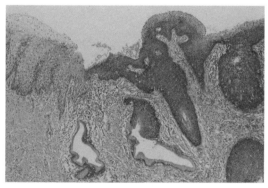

42. This is a slide of a cervix.

a. What does it show?
b. Is there evidence of invasion?
c. If the lesion was completely excised by cone biopsy what follow-up would you arrange?
d. Prior to treatment what would you anticipate the smear on this woman to reveal?

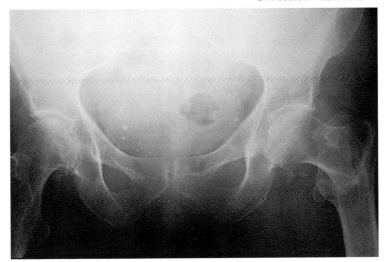

43.

a. What does this photograph show?
b. Name the probable underlying pathology.
c. What other sites are affected by the underlying pathology?
d. What are the causes of the underlying problem?
e. What are the long-term implications for this woman's health?

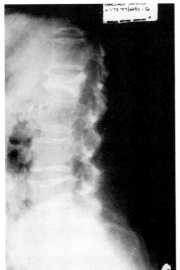

44.

a. What are the two diagnoses present?
b. What are the usual symptoms?
c. What are the risk factors for the underlying disease?
d. What type of bone predominates in the spine?
e. What are the lifestyle implications for the conditions illustrated?

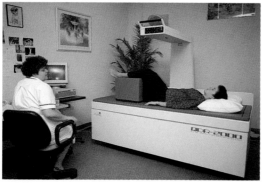

45.

a. What is this examination?
b. At what age does a woman attain peak bone mass?
c. What measures can help to maximize the peak bone mass?
d. What is the age-related rate of bone loss?
e. What is the rate of bone loss following the menopause?

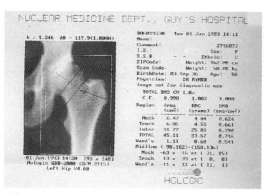

46.

a. How was this image produced?
b. What is being measured?
c. What other tests are available to obtain this measurement?
d. What is Ward's triangle?
e. What are the advantages of this test over the other methods?

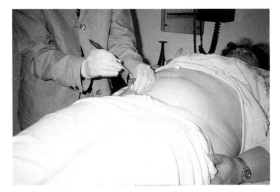

47.

a. What is the procedure that is being performed?
b. What is the likely ingredient?
c. Why are these administered?
d. How often are they administered?
e. Should progestogens be given as well?

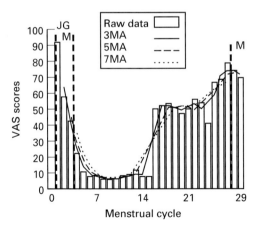

48. These scores relate to a woman who suffers from the premenstrual syndrome.

a. How would you define this syndrome?
b. What are some typical symptoms?
c. How is the condition diagnosed?
d. What treatment modalities are available?

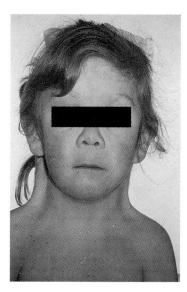

49.

a. What is this condition?
b. What is the characteristic karyotype?
c. What are the typical physical findings?
d. Is spontaneous pregnancy a possibility for this person?
e. How can this condition be diagnosed antenatally?

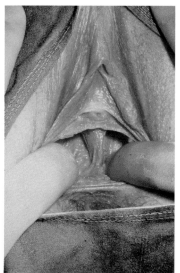

50.

a. Name this congenital abnormality.
b. Describe the embryological basis.
c. What gynaecological symptoms may this cause?
d. With what other abnormalities may this condition be associated?
e. What possible problems may this cause in labour?

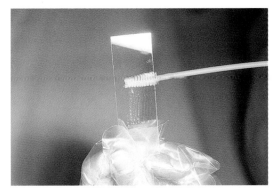

51.

a. What is the name of this instrument?
b. What area does it sample?
c. When would you use this?

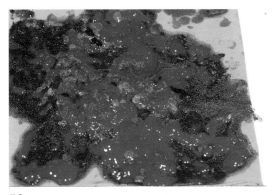

52. This tissue was removed at a D&C.

a. What does this illustrate?
b. What is the diagnosis?
c. What are the typical symptoms?
d. What are the signs?
e. What is the management?

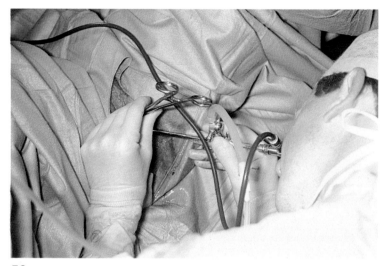

53. This woman presented with postmenopausal bleeding.

a. What investigation is being performed?
b. What is being passed through the rubber tubing?
c. What does this operation enable you to do?

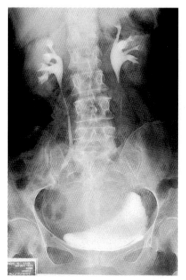

54.

a. What investigation has been performed?
b. Describe the findings.
c. With what urinary symptoms may this patient present?
d. What gynaecological causes may result in this picture?

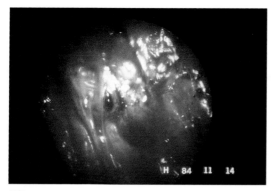

55.

a. What is the diagnosis?
b. What are the common sites affected?
c. What modalities of treatment are available?
d. Can hormonal replacement therapy (HRT) be prescribed to women with a past history of this condition?

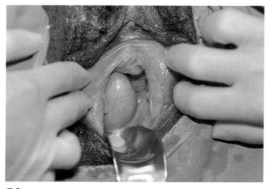

56.

a. What is the diagnosis?
b. What is the differential diagnosis?
c. What are typical presenting symptoms?
d. What is the treatment?

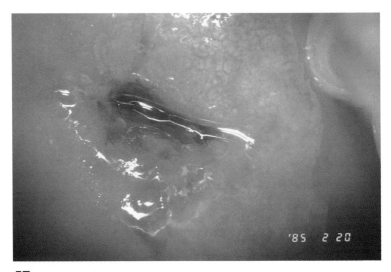

57.

a. What solution has been used on the cervix?
b. What can you see?
c. Do you think this is a severe or a minor lesion?
d. A biopsy showed CIN 1. Describe CIN 1.
e. Can spontaneous regression occur?

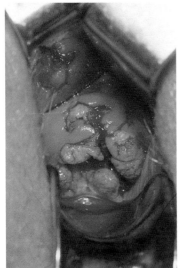

58. This woman complained of continual loss of fluid per vagina.

a. Describe the findings.
b. What is the diagnosis?
c. Define this condition.
d. What are the common causes?
e. What are the principles of management?

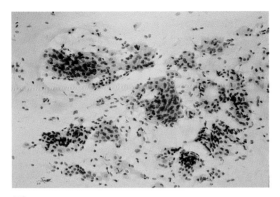

59. This is a cytological slide of a vaginal smear.

a. What is the morphology of normal vaginal epithelial cells?
b. What factors contribute to a healthy vaginal environment?

This slide illustrates an atrophic pattern.

c. In what situations may this pattern be seen?

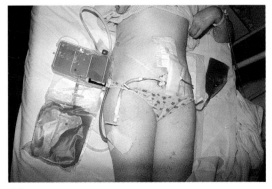

60.

a. What bladder drainage is being used here?
b. What other drain is present?
c. What incisions are evident?
d. What are the advantages of this form of bladder drainage?

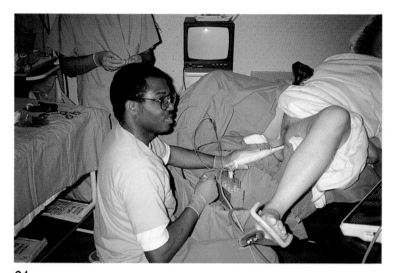

61. This woman is undergoing oocyte retrieval in an in-vitro fertilization treatment cycle.

a. What methods are available for oocyte retrieval?
b. What treatment generally precedes this procedure?
c. What was the original indication for IVF?
d. What further indications have been added more recently?

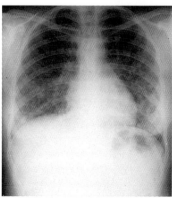

62. This young woman was seen with metastatic choriocarcinoma.

a. What is the incidence of metastatic disease after molar evacuation?
b. What is the main route of spread?
c. What are the common metastatic sites?
d. How should this patient be evaluated?
e. Which factors affect the prognosis?

Semen analysis report

Normal values for our laboratory are given in brackets: they are based on specimens received within 1 hour of ejaculation and produced after 3 to 5 days of abstinence.

Clinical data: Subfertility Investigation

Patient DOB: 24/12/49

Time produced: 10:10 hr   **Time at lab:** 10:15 hr

Abstinence: 6 days   **Volume:** 2.5ml (normal 2–5 ml)

pH: 7.5 (normal 7.2–7.8)

Sperm count: 67 million/ml (normal 20–300 million/ml)

Sperm motility (more than 50% should be motile after 1 hr)
75% at start
70% after 1 hr

Sperm morphology (less than 50% abnormal forms should be present)
58% normal forms
42% abnormal forms

63.

a. Is this result normal or abnormal?
b. What instructions would you give for collection?
c. What is a postcoital test?
d. Explain a positive and negative postcoital test.

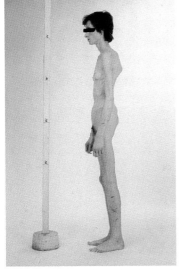

64. This patient presented with secondary amenorrhoea.

a. Define secondary amenorrhoea.
b. Divide the causes of amenorrhoea into anatomical compartments.
c. What is the likely cause in this patient? What compartment is affected?
d. What baseline investigations would you perform?

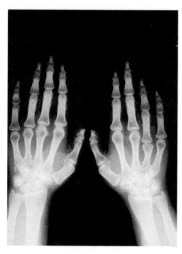

65.

a. What is this examination?
b. What is the abnormality?
c. This patient has Turner's syndrome; what would the karyotype be?
d. What are other clinical features of this syndrome?

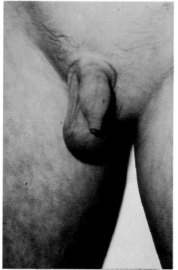

66.

a. What abnormality does this show?
b. Are these more common in term or preterm infants?
c. If this condition is discovered at birth what is the management?
d. Could this patient suffer from male infertility?

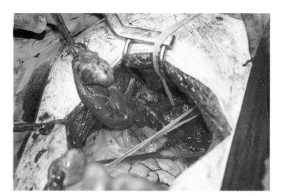

67. The illustrations in questions 67 and 68 relate to Wertheim's hysterectomy.

a. What two options are available for the first line treatment of cervical carcinoma?
b. What factors determine the choice of treatment?
c. What structures are removed?
d. What structures have been isolated by the uppermost and lowermost tapes?

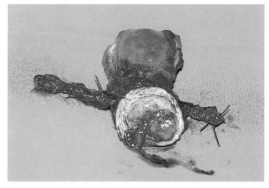

68.

a. What are the indications for a Wertheim's hysterectomy?
b. What lymph node groups are dissected during the procedure?
c. What are the complications of a Wertheim's hysterectomy?
d. What are the relative merits of the surgical approach and radiation therapy?

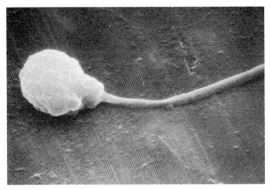

69.

a. What does this electron scanning micrograph illustrate?
b. What are the structural components?
c. Where is this structure produced?
d. What is the stimulus for its production?
e. What is the function of the Leydig cells?

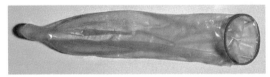

70.

a. What is the failure rate of condoms?
b. Describe the method of application and removal.
c. What are the advantages of this device?
d. If this device 'bursts', what is the management?

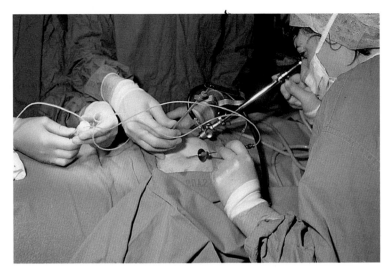

71.

a. What assisted conception technique is being performed?
b. Describe the technique.
c. What are the indications for this technique?
d. How is the patient monitored prior to the technique?

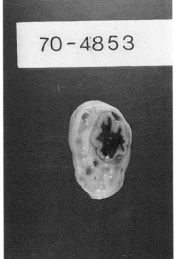

72.

a. What is this structure?
b. Which hormone is thought to exert a luteotrophic effect on this structure?
c. At what stage of pregnancy does the level of this luteotrophic hormone begin to fall?
d. What hormones does this structure secrete in pregnancy?
e. At what gestation will removal of the above structure usually result in spontaneous abortion?

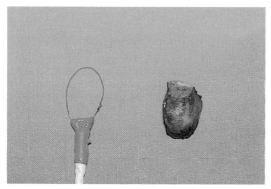

73.

a. What is the name of this specimen and instrument?
b. What is the purpose of this procedure?
c. What investigations should precede this procedure?
d. What alternative procedures are available?
e. What complications can follow this procedure and what advice would you give to the patient?

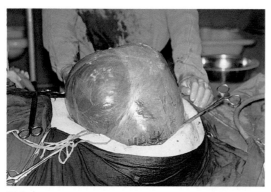

74. This abdominal mass was removed from an elderly woman.

a. With what symptoms may this woman have presented?
b. On examination, what signs would help with the differential diagnosis?
c. What investigations would you order?
d. How is the definitive diagnosis made?
e. What is the most likely gynaecological diagnosis?

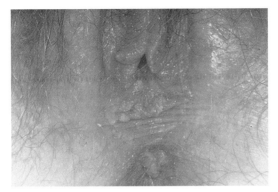

75.

a. What term describes this appearance?
b. What is the aetiological agent?
c. How is this condition usually acquired?
d. What modes of therapy are available?
e. How would you counsel this patient following treatment?

Semen analysis report

Normal values for our laboratory are given in brackets: they are based on specimens received within 1 hour of ejaculation and produced after 3 to 5 days of abstinence.

Clinical data: Subfertility Investigation

Patient DOB: 20/10/53

Time produced: 08:30 hr   **Time at lab:** 09:15 hr

Abstinence: 3 days   **Volume:** 3.0 ml (normal 2–5 ml)

pH: 7.5 (normal 7.2–7.8)

Sperm count: 2 million/ml (normal 20–300 million/ml)

Sperm motility (more than 50% should be motile after 1 hr)
65% at start
65% after 1 hr

Sperm morphology (less than 50% abnormal forms should be present)
68% normal forms
32% abnormal forms

76.

a. What does this result show?
b. What history would you elicit from the donor?
c. What further investigations would you do?
d. What treatment would you offer?

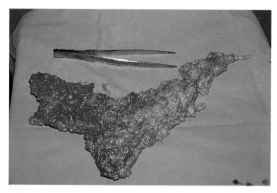

77. This specimen was removed at omentectomy.

a. What was the likely primary medical condition?
b. What is the typical pattern of spread of the primary condition?
c. Why was the above specimen removed?
d. What factors influence the prognosis of the primary condition?

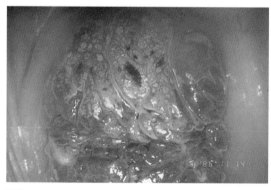

78.

a. This cervix has been stained with acetic acid. Describe what you see.
b. What does this colposcopic appearance suggest?
c. What would be your management?
d. Can these changes spontaneously revert to normal?

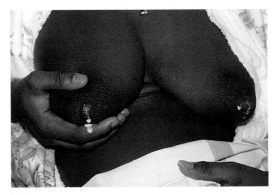

79.

a. Describe what you see.
b. What is this condition called?
c. What gynaecological condition may she have presented with?
d. What investigations would you perform?

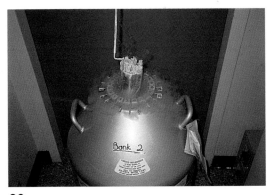

80. These are tubes of stored frozen semen.

a. How are these tubes stored?
b. How are semen donors screened?
c. What are the indications for donor insemination?

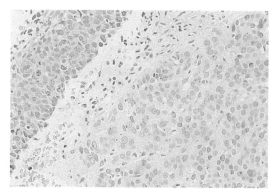

81. This histology slide shows a section of cervix.

a. What can you see?
b. What operation should be performed?
c. Could this woman have HRT when she is postmenopausal?

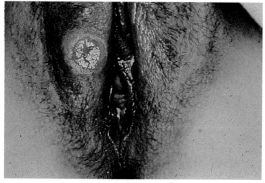

82.

a. What is the diagnosis?
b. Name the causative organism.
c. At what time does the illustrated lesion develop?
d. How is the definitive diagnosis made?
e. How should the illustrated condition be managed?

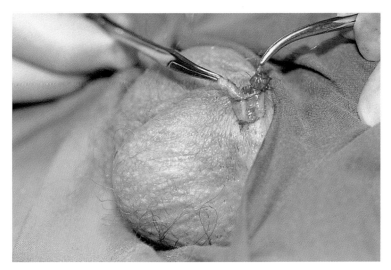

83.

a. What structure has been isolated?
b. What is the name of this operation?
c. What issues should be discussed in the preoperative counselling?
d. What are the complications of this operation?

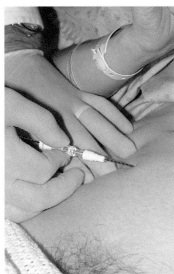

84. This woman is being given a GnRH agonist as part of her treatment for uterine fibroids.

a. How do GnRH agonists exert their effects?
b. What are the possible routes of administration?
c. What is the effect of these medications on fibroids?
d. What are the other clinical uses of GnRH agonists in gynaecology?
e. What are the side-effects (short- and longterm)?

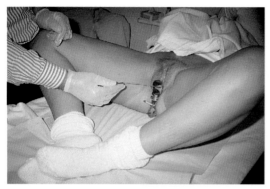

85.

a. What is the nature and purpose of this procedure?
b. What analgesia is required?
c. What are the contraindications?
d. How is this procedure performed?
e. What are the possible adverse reactions?

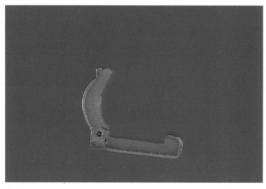

86.

a. What is this?
b. What is it used for?
c. How would you counsel the patient prior to the procedure?
d. What is the failure rate?

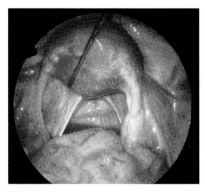

87.

a. What structure is the probe supporting?
b. What are the white band-like structures in the centre portion of the photograph?
c. Is the free fluid that is seen necessarily pathological?
d. What structure occupies the posterior one-third of the illustration?

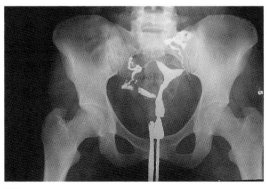

88.

a. What is this investigation?
b. What are the indications for this investigation?
c. What are the risks of this procedure?
d. What does this investigation show?

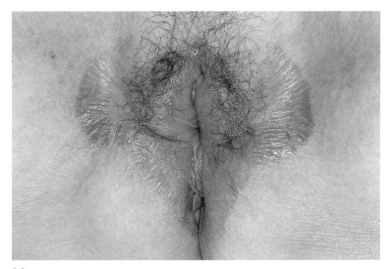

89. This woman presented with pruritus vulvae.

a. What are the possible causes?
b. How are non-neoplastic vulval epithelial disorders classified?
c. What investigation is required prior to treatment?
d. What is the treatment of the two common forms of 'vulval dystrophy'?

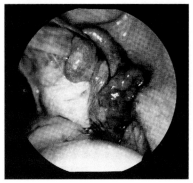

90.

a. What operation has been performed?
b. What are the main indications for this procedure?
c. What are the relative merits for this procedure in comparison to hysterosalpingography?
d. What comment would you make concerning this patient's tubes?

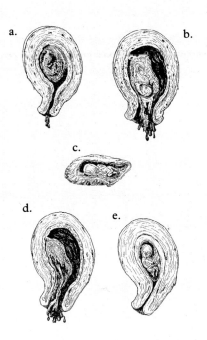

91.

a.–e. Name the five types of spontaneous abortions.

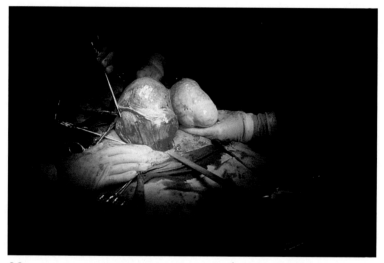

92. This woman presented with a large pelvic mass.

a. What is the diagnosis?
b. Is the mass on the left of the uterus likely to be benign or malignant?
c. This woman is 54. What operation is being performed?

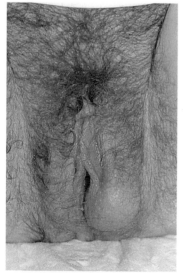

93.

a. Describe the physical findings.
b. What is the most likely diagnosis?
c. How does this lesion form?
d. What complication can occur?
e. How should this patient be managed?

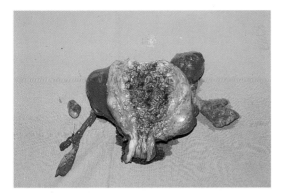

94. **This woman presented with postmenopausal bleeding.**

a. What is the diagnosis?
b. List the typical risk factors.
c. How is the diagnosis usually confirmed?
d. What is the typical histology of this lesion?
e. What are the characteristic patterns of spread?
f. What are the principles of management?

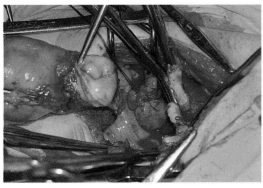

95.

a. What operation is being performed?
b. Have the ovaries been removed?
c. Was the vagina prepared with any solution?
d. What suture has been used to tie the pedicles?

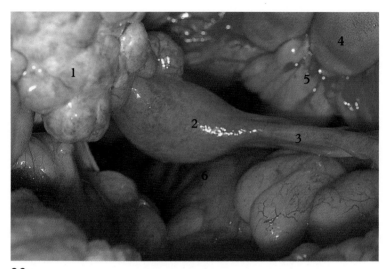

96. This woman has a left ovarian fibroma. Name the structures that are numbered 1 to 6.

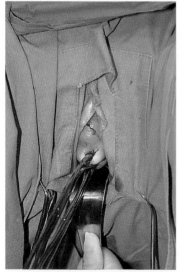

97.

a. Describe what you see.
b. Name the instruments illustrated.
c. What is the classification of this disorder?
d. What aetiological factors contribute to this condition?
e. What are the typical presenting symptoms?

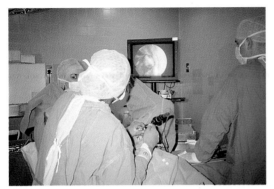

98.

a. What operation is being performed?
b. What are the advantages of using a television screen?

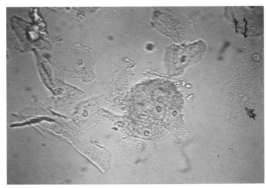

99.

a. What is the commonest cause of vaginitis?
b. What clue is present in the illustrated Gram stain?
c. What is the composition of the clue?
d. Describe the typical resultant vaginal discharge.
e. How should this vaginitis be treated?

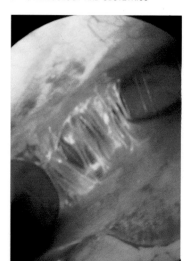

100. These adhesions were noted between the liver and anterior parietal peritoneum.

a. What is the name of this condition?
b. What is the aetiology?
c. What is the infective organism?
d. How does this condition usually present in gynaecology?
e. What is the treatment?

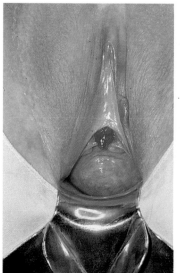

101.

a. What is the bulging structure?
b. What structure underlies the bulging tissue?
c. With what symptoms may this patient have presented?
d. What operation will correct this abnormality?
e. What urethral abnormality is evident?

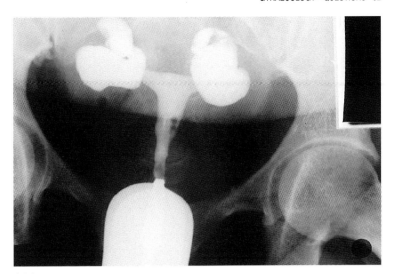

102.

a. What does this hysterosalpingogram reveal?
b. What is the most likely cause?
c. At what level is the blockage present?
d. If infertility is the patient's main concern what treatment options are available?

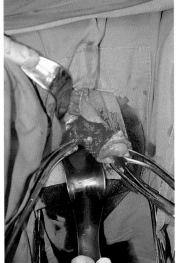

103.

a. What operation is being performed?
b. What are the supporting structures of the uterus?
c. What surrounding structures are at risk of damage during this procedure?
d. What complications can occur postoperatively?

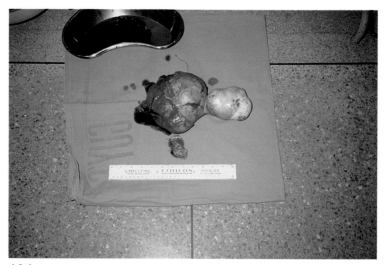

104. This is a postoperative specimen.

a. What is the specimen?
b. How may this patient have presented?
c. Why has the cervix been removed separately?
d. If this woman had been under 40 years, would her ovaries have been conserved or removed in the absence of other risk factors?

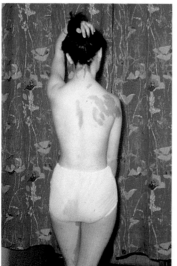

105. This girl has precocious puberty.

a. Describe what you see.
b. What are these lesions called?
c. What is the pathology behind this condition?
d. What is the diagnosis?

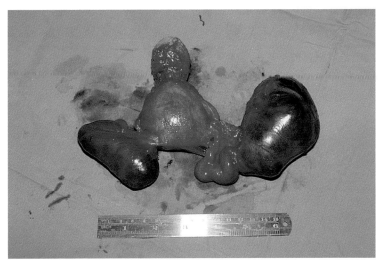

106.

a. Describe what you see.
b. The diagnosis is bilateral haemotosalpinges. How may she have presented and what are possible pathologies?
c. Is the uterus normal size?
d. Has she had a total or a subtotal hysterectomy?

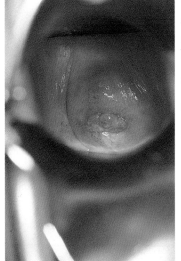

107. This lesion was present in a postmenopausal woman.

a. What is the diagnosis?
b. What is the most likely presenting symptom?
c. What is the typical histology of this lesion?
d. How would you manage this patient?
e. How would you manage this lesion in a young woman?

Obstetrics—Questions

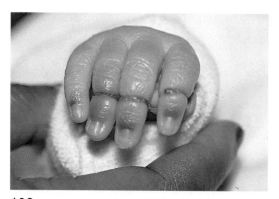

108. **This is a hand of a newborn baby.**

a. What can you see?
b. How do these occur?
c. What is the prognosis?

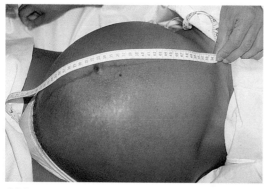

109.

a. What are the causes of a woman being supposedly 'large for dates'?
b. Describe your method of assessing such a patient.

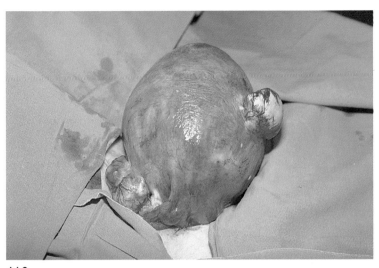

110. These structures were noted at caesarean section.

a. What are they and what complications can they cause in pregnancy?
b. What complications can they cause in labour and immediately post delivery?
c. How should they be dealt with at caesarean section?

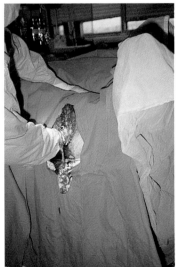

111.

a. What procedure is being performed?
b. What are the preoperative requirements?
c. What risks does this procedure entail?
d. What factors predispose to a retained placenta?

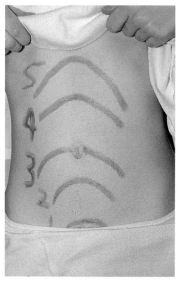

112. **What gestations are compatible with each of the markings illustrated?**

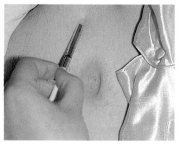

113. **This woman has insulin-dependent diabetes in pregnancy.**

a. What are the fetal risks?
b. What are the maternal risks?
c. What is the antenatal management?
d. What neonatal problems can be anticipated?
e. How would you counsel this patient post delivery?

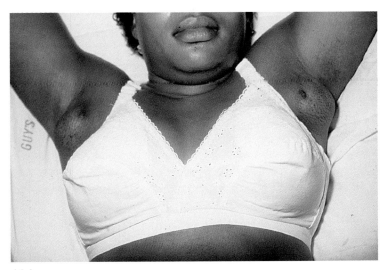

114. This woman is at 30 weeks' gestation.

a. What is the most likely diagnosis and what symptoms may this cause?
b. Where are accessory nipples normally found?
c. What is the natural history of these lumps post partum?
d. How can the lumps be suppressed post partum and is surgery indicated?

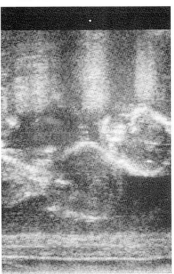

115.

a. What is the diagnosis?
b. What is the incidence?
c: What factors are contributing to a change in the incidence of this condition?
d. What antenatal care will you offer this patient?
e. What complications can occur in the first trimester?

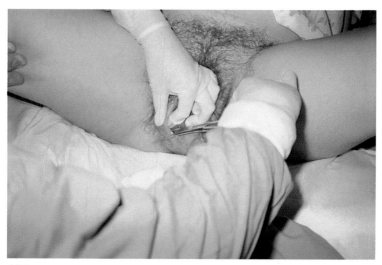

116.

a. What operation is being performed?
b. What is the purpose of this operation?
c. What are the disadvantages of this procedure?
d. What different incisions may be performed?

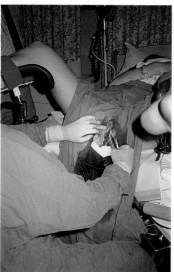

117.

a. What is the technique for performing a mediolateral episiotomy?
b. Which tissues are cut?
c. What are the principles of repair?

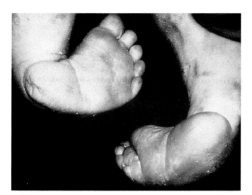

118.

a. What is the term for this very characteristic appearance?
b. If diagnosed antenatally what is the significance of this finding?
c. What nongenetic causes can result in this appearance?

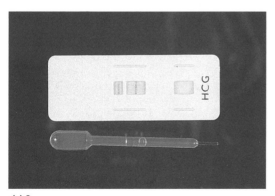

119.

a. What is this test?
b. How is the test conducted?
c. How do you read the result?
d. For how long is the result stable?
e. What is the sensitivity of the test?
f. How soon can the condition being sought be diagnosed with this test?

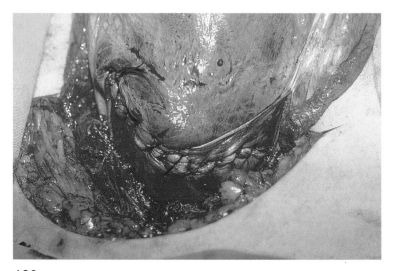

120.

a. What operation has been performed?
b. What layers are incised during this operation?
c. What early postoperative complications can occur?
d. What late postoperative complications can occur?

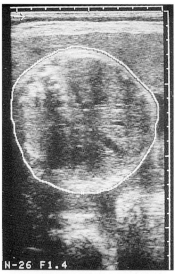

121.

a. What is being measured?
b. At what level should this measurement be taken?
c. What is the purpose of this measurement?
d. What structures can usually be confidently identified within the prescribed area?

Department of Clinical Chemistry	
Jane Smith	Date of birth: 20/10/54
Investigations: Urinalysis	
Specimen date and time: 12/12/93	15:00

Timed urine	24 hr collection
Protein	3.0 g/1
Volume	2315 ml
Protein	6.9 g/spec

122. This woman is at 33 weeks' gestation, weight 70 kg.

a. What is the normal daily urinary excretion of protein?
b. What are the possible diagnoses?
c. What is the minimum hourly urine output you would accept?
d. What would you expect this woman's urinary output to be?

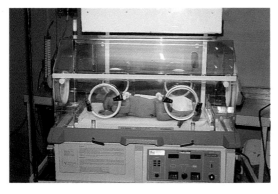

123.

a. What treatment is this neonate undergoing?
b. What is the incidence of neonatal jaundice? What factors contribute to physiological jaundice?
c. What are the causes of neonatal jaundice?
d. Which clinical criteria would suggest the presence of a nonphysiological cause?

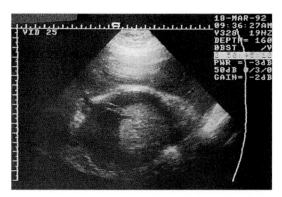

124. Fetal ascites due to rhesus isoimmunization.

a. How is this disease screened for in the antenatal clinic?
b. If antibodies are detected what is the management?
c. By what test can the number of fetal cells in the maternal circulation be determined?

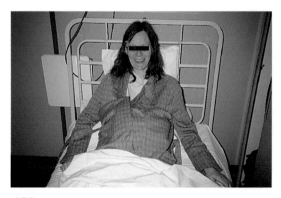

125. This pregnant woman has had six children.

a. What obstetric term can be applied to this woman?
b. What are the potential risks of this condition?
c. What particular precautions are required in labour?
d. How would you counsel this woman post-delivery?

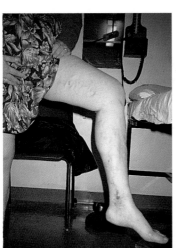

126.

a. What is the diagnosis?
b. What other sites may be affected in pregnancy?
c. What are the contributory aetiological factors?
d. What are the usual symptoms?
e. What complications can occur?
f. What advice would you give this woman?

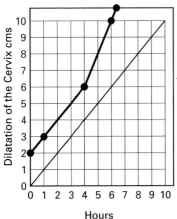

127.

a. What is this graph called?
b. What is its purpose?
c. How would you describe the progress?
d. What is the expected cervical dilatation in labour?
e. What are the components of normal labour progress?

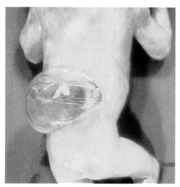

128.

a. How does this lesion result?
b. How can this condition be diagnosed antenatally?
c. What is the prognosis?
d. What dietary advice should all potential mothers now receive?

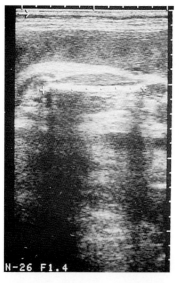

129.

a. What part of the fetal femur is being measured?
b. Are the proximal or distal fetal limb bones easier to image?
c. From what gestation can the femur length be routinely measured?
d. Of what use is this measurement?

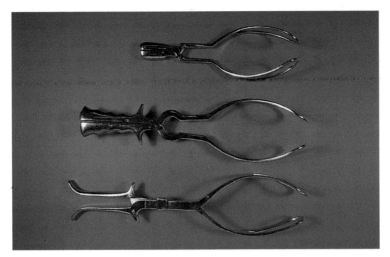

130.

a. What are these instruments and name each type?
b. Name the component parts.
c. What are the differences between the lower two instruments?
d. What is asynclitism and which of these instruments can correct it?
e. What functions are performed?

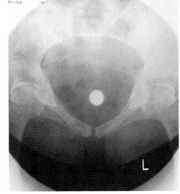

131.

a. What type of pelvis is illustrated?
b. What is the incidence of this type of pelvis in the female population?
c. What are the salient features of this type of pelvis?
d. What is the effect on labour?

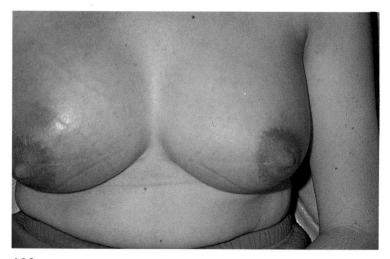

132. This woman has an erythematous hot fluctuant area to the left of her right nipple.

a. What is the diagnosis?
b. What is the usual aetiology?
c. How should this condition be treated?

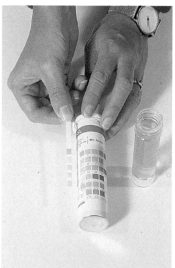

133.

a. At what time was this procedure performed?
b. What is being tested?
c. Is this result normal?
d. What is the place of this investigation in the antenatal clinic?
e. Can this sample be used for microbiological assessment?

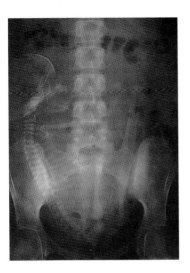

134.

a. What is the diagnosis?
b. What factors are associated with this presentation?
c. Name the different types of this presentation.
d. What is the incidence of this presentation?
e. What are the management options available for this woman at 37 weeks' gestation?

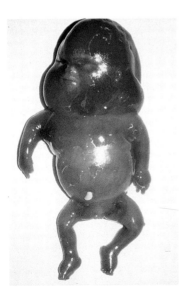

135.

a. What very obvious abnormality is present in this fetus?
b. What is the nature of this problem?
c. What is the incidence of associated chromosomal abnormalities?
d. What is the classic chromosomal abnormality found?
e. What is the prognosis?

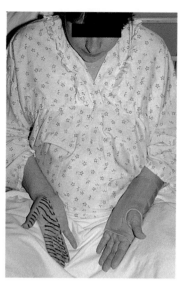

136. This patient is at 38 weeks' gestation.

a. What is the diagnosis?
b. What are the usual symptoms?
c. What is the neurological basis of this disorder?
d. What aetiological factor results in this disorder in pregnancy?
e. How may this patient be helped?

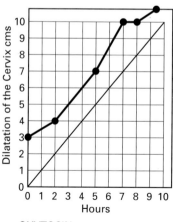

OXYTOCIN

137.

a. Describe the progress of this labour.
b. What are the possible causes of the lack of progress depicted?
c. What remedial action was taken?
d. What was the outcome?
e. Would this management be acceptable in a multiparous patient?

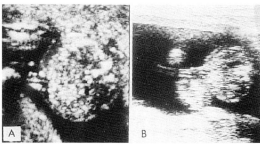

138.

a. What abnormality is evident in B?
b. Define this condition.
c. What are the differentiating features of this condition?
d. What is the incidence of associated congenital abnormalities?
e. What is the management and prognosis of this disorder?

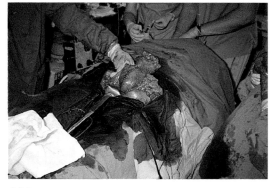

139.

a. What type of caesarean section has been performed?
b. What structure is at the cephalad aspect of the uterus?
c. How many suture layers are used in this uterine closure?
d. What type of delivery should this woman have next time?

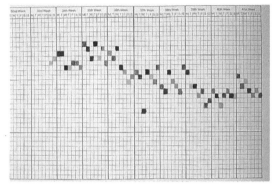

140.

a. What is being illustrated?
b. How would you instruct a patient with regard to this chart?
c. Is this chart normal or abnormal?
d. What action should be taken in the presence of an abnormal chart?
e. At what gestation are fetal movements initially felt?

Haematology report	
Jane Doe	**Date of birth: 12/3/61**
Investigations: FBC	
Neutrophils	$2.89 \times 10^9/1$
Lymphocytes	$1.68 \times 10^9/1$
Monocytes	$0.24 \times 10^9/1$
Eosinophils	$0.16 \times 10^9/1$
Basophils	$0.02 \times 10^9/1$
RBC $\times 10^{12}/1$	4.69
Hct	0.402
MCV fl	85.7
MCH pg	29.9
MCHC g/dl	34.8
WBC $\times 10^9/1$	4.99
Hb g/dl	14.0
Plts $\times 10^9/1$	43

141. This result is from a woman who is 32 weeks pregnant.

a. What do these results indicate?
b. What is the most likely diagnosis?
c. The 24h urine result is 6 g per day. What is your management?
d. What is the normal haematocrit in pregnancy?

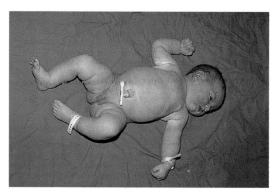

142.

a. What is the descriptive term for the size of this newborn baby?
b. What is the classic maternal predisposing cause?
c. What problems can be encountered in labour?
d. If diagnosed antenatally, what precautions should be taken?

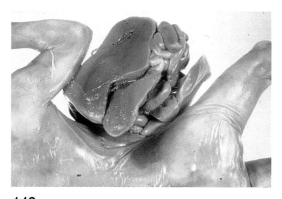

143. This fetus has an omphalocoele.

a. Define this condition.
b. What structures may be contained within an omphalocoele?
c. What is the incidence of associated anomalies?
d. What is the prognosis?
e. What is the obstetrical management?

Glucose tolerance test	
Jane Smith 28 weeks pregnant 100 g glucose load	**Date of birth: 24/4/64**
Time	**Plasma glucose**
Fasting	6.4 mmol/1
1 hour	13.2 mmol/1
2 hour	11.3 mmol/1
3 hour	9.2 mmol/1

144.

a. This woman has no history of diabetes. What is the diagnosis?
b. What is the definition of this diagnosis?
c. How does carbohydrate metabolism change during pregnancy?
d. What is the management of this condition?
e. What are the longterm implications of this condition?

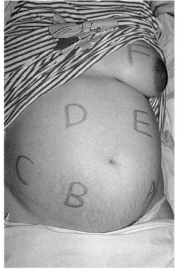

145. Where will the fetal heart best be heard in the following fetal presentations/positions?

a. Breech, right sacro-anterior.
b. Cephalic, left occipito-posterior.
c. Cephalic, right occipito-posterior.
d. Breech, left sacro-anterior.
e. Cephalic, right occipito-anterior.
f. In what position will the fetal heart best be heard in position F?

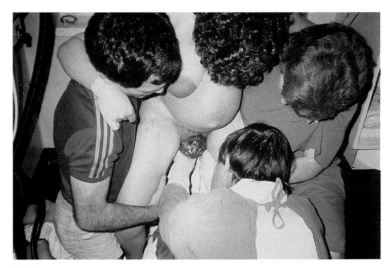

146. This woman is undergoing a normal vaginal delivery.

a. How is labour diagnosed? What positions are used for delivery?
b. Describe the normal mechanism for delivery for a fetus that presents cephalically in position left occipito-anterior.
c. What is the incidence of cord around the neck?
d. How do you deal with this situation?

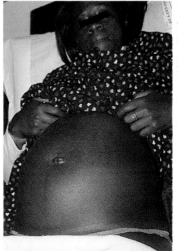

147. This woman was seen in the antenatal clinic at 37 weeks' gestation with a transverse lie.

a. Define transverse lie.
b. What are the predisposing factors?
c. What are the risks associated with this condition?
d. How should this woman be managed?

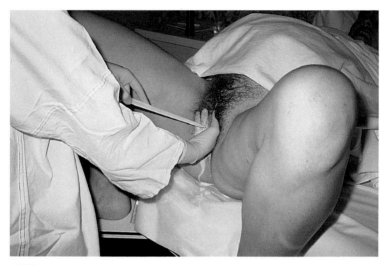

148.

a. How would you define induction of labour?
b. What conditions must be present before an induction of labour is performed?
c. What are the contraindications to artificial rupture of membranes?
d. What complications can arise following induction of labour?

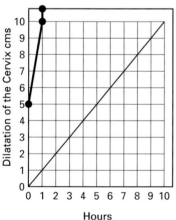

Dilatation of the Cervix cms

Hours

149.

a. What term describes this labour?
b. What is the definition of this term?
c. What are the causes of this condition?
d. In what situations does this occur?
e. What are the potential risks of this type of labour?

150.

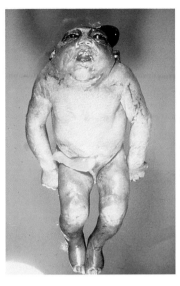

a. What congenital abnormality is illustrated?
b. How would you define this disorder?
c. How is this condition usually diagnosed?
d. What is unusual about this photograph?
e. What are common associated congenital abnormalities?
f. What is the prognosis?

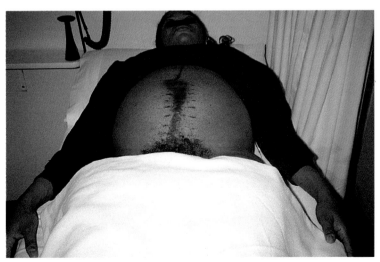

151. This woman has had a previous classical caesarean section.

a. What are the modern indications for this operation?
b. What are the disadvantages of a classical caesarean section?
c. How should this woman be delivered in her current pregnancy?

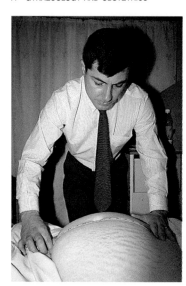

152.

a. How is the symphysio–fundal height measured?
b. Define the fetal lie.
c. How can cephalic and breech presentations be distinguished clinically?
d. Define engagement.
e. What is meant by the term 'fetal position'?

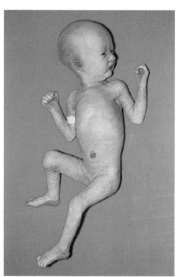

153.

a. This infant shows evidence of which clinical disorder?
b. What are the typical clinical features?
c. What problems may this infant face in the early neonatal period?
d. What is the longterm prognosis for this infant?

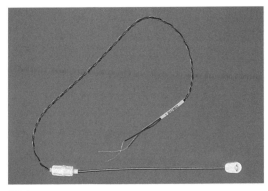

154.

a. What is this device?
b. What is its purpose?
c. What is the method of application?
d. How is the signal generated?
e. What are the potential complications associated with its use?

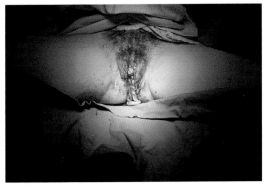

155.

a. What obstetric catastrophe has occurred?
b. What are the predisposing factors?
c. How is the diagnosis usually made?
d. What is the management?

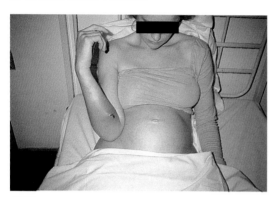

156.

a. What obvious problem is evident in this pregnant woman?
b. What is the most likely predisposing factor?
c. What pregnancy complications may occur in this woman?
d. How should this woman be managed?

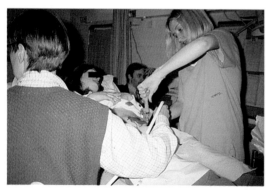

157. **The woman in the slide is 16 weeks pregnant.**

a. What procedure is being performed?
b. What is the woman on the left holding in her right hand?
c. Why is this test performed?
d. What is the risk of the procedure to the pregnancy?
e. What alternative test can be offered at an earlier gestation?

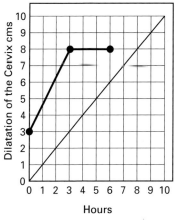

Hours

158. **This is a multiparous woman.**

a. Describe what has occurred.
b. What is this situation called?
c. What are the causes?
d. What would be the typical cause if this was a primigravid woman?
e. What is the management of this multiparous patient?

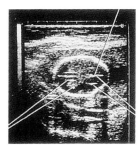

159.

a. What view has been obtained?
b. What parameter is widely used in the estimation of gestational age?
c. What is the accuracy of this parameter?
d. What is the significance of choroid plexus cysts?

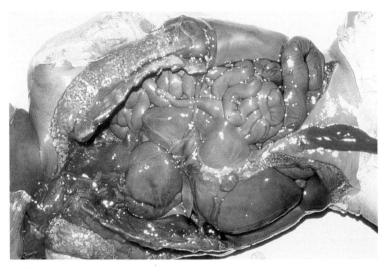

160.

a. What is the name of this disorder?
b. If diagnosed antenatally what are the typical ultrasound findings?
c. What is the incidence of concomitant anomalies?
d. What is the prognosis?
e. What is the obstetrical management of this condition?

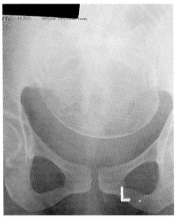

161. This fetal head is unengaged late in pregnancy.

a. At what gestation does the fetal head engage in a primigravid woman?
b. What factors may prevent engagement?
c. At 40 weeks, how would you manage this woman?

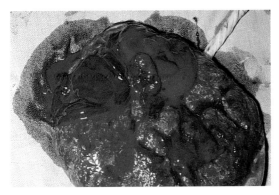

162.

a. What are the causes of antepartum haemorrhage?
b. Which cause is evident in this illustration?
c. How does this problem usually present?
d. Which signs would typically be present on examination?
e. What complications may be seen?
f. How should this condition be managed?

Haematology report	
Jane Smith **Investigations:** FBC	**Date of birth:** 12/8/64
Ferritin	11.0 µg/1 (15–20)
Vitamin B12	293.8 µg/1 (200–900)
Serum folate	2.3 µg/1 (2.0–20.2)
RBC × 10¹²/1	3.08
Hct	.228
MCV fl	74.0
MCH pg	22.7
MCHC g/dl	30.7
WBC × 10⁹/1	8.88
Hb g/dl	7.0
Plts × 10⁹/1	81

163. These results are from a woman who is 30 weeks pregnant.

a. What is the diagnosis?
b. What is the most common cause?
c. How would you treat this patient?
d. How do you check for treatment response?
e. What treatment options are available for this patient at 40 weeks gestation?

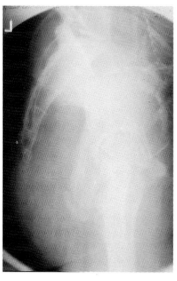

164.

a. What is this investigation?
b. What information can be obtained?
c. What measurements are usually recorded?
d. When would you order this investigation?
e. By what other means can pelvic size be assessed?

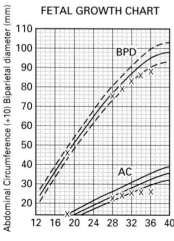

FETAL GROWTH CHART

Abdominal Circumference (÷10) Biparietal diameter (mm)

BPD

AC

12 16 20 24 28 32 36 40

165.

a. Explain this graph. What does it depict?
b. What is the diagnosis?
c. What is the definition of the diagnosis and name the two types?
d. What are the aetiological factors?
e. What is the management of the situation depicted? Justify your answer.

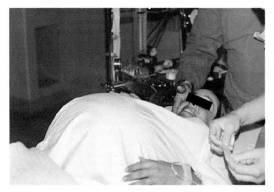

166. The woman illustrated is about to have a general anaesthetic for an emergency caesarean section.

a. What problems associated with general anaesthesia can occur?
b. What are the reasons for this increased risk?
c. What can be given preoperatively to reduce this risk?

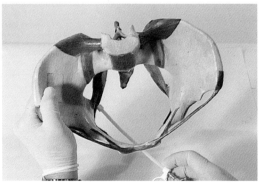

167.

a. What procedure is being simulated?
b. What is the purpose of this procedure?
c. What is the relevant anatomy?
d. In what situations is this procedure used?
e. What precaution should be taken in the performance of this procedure?

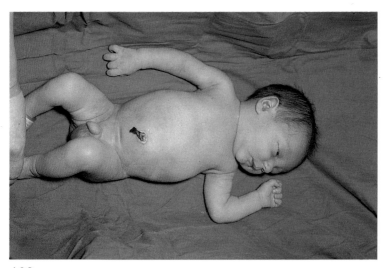

168.

a. What is the diagnosis?
b. By what colloquialism is this otherwise known?
c. How does this injury occur?
d. What is the neurological basis of this disorder?
e. What is the prognosis?

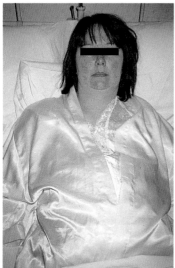

169.

a. What medical condition is evident in this pregnant woman?
b. What is the effect of this condition on pregnancy?
c. What is the effect of pregnancy on the course of the condition?
d. Outline the management principles.

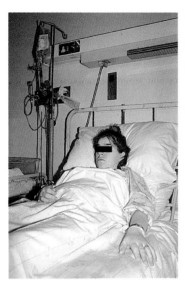

170.

a. What is being infused into this woman?
b. This woman had the problem of uterine atony.
   How would you manage it?
c. What are the complications of blood transfusions?

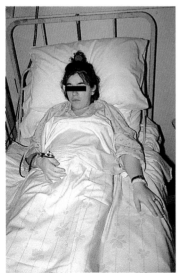

171.

a. This woman has had a primary postpartum haemorrhage. What is the definition?
b. What is the incidence of postpartum haemorrhage?
c. What are the causes?
d. What is your immediate management of a postpartum haemorrhage?

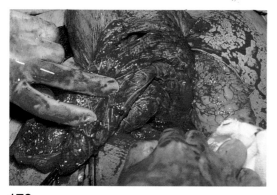

172. This is a picture of a caesarean section and the baby has been delivered.

a. What appears to be the problem?
b. This woman had a previous caesarean section and in this pregnancy had a placenta praevia. Could this complication have been predicted?
c. What is the management?

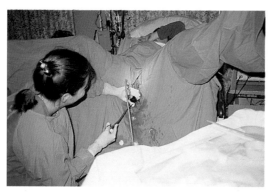

173.

a. What procedure is being performed?
b. What are the contraindications to this procedure?
c. What complications can occur to the fetus?
d. What sample is obtained with this procedure?
e. Concerning the result obtained, state the generally accepted normal range.

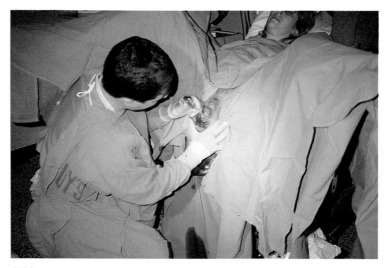

174.

a. What operation is being performed and what are the indications?
b. What conditions must be present before embarking upon this procedure?
c. What are the potential complications?

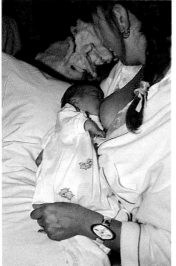

175.

a. How is lactation initiated in the puerperium?
b. What is the composition of human breast milk?
c. What are the advantages of breast milk and breastfeeding?

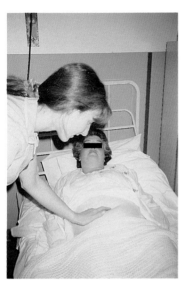

176. The woman illustrated had delivered a 3.5-kg term infant 12 hours previously.

a. What is the midwife doing?
b. If the fundus was above the umbilicus what would the midwife suspect?
c. If the woman has not passed urine since delivery what action would the midwife take?

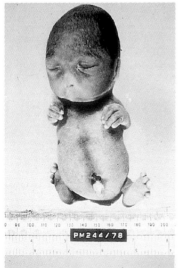

177.

a. What is this condition?
b. What is the definition of this disorder?
c. What is the cause?
d. What is amelia?

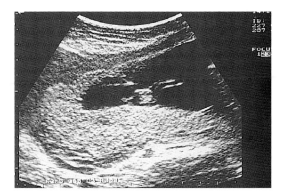

178. **This photograph was taken during a cordocentesis procedure. The point of the needle is about to enter the umbilical cord.**

a. What is the purpose of this test?
b. By what other means may an appropriate specimen be obtained?
c. What are the indications?
d. What are the risks?

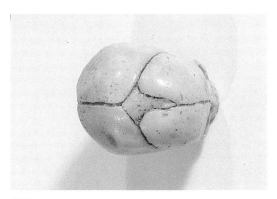

179.

a. Name the sutures and fontanelle that are demonstrated on this specimen.
b. Define the terms vertex and bregma.
c. What diameter presents in a normal labour with a flexed fetal head?
d. Define denominator. What is the denominator for cephalic, breech and face presentations?

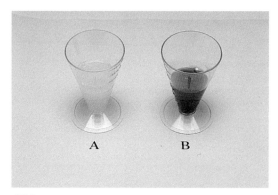

180. These are two examples of liquor.

a. What accounts for the appearance of sample B?
b. If sample B was obtained following rupture of the membranes in labour, what would be your management?
c. In the presence of liquor such as B, what special precautions are required at delivery?

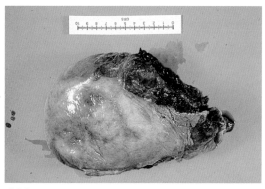

181.

a. What is this specimen?
b. What aetiological factors result in this obstetric catastrophe?
c. What are the clinical features?
d. What is the management of this condition?

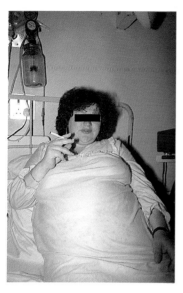

182. This woman is at 37 weeks' gestation.

a. What is she doing wrong?
b. What are the potential harmful effects of this habit in pregnancy?
c. By what mechanisms does this habit exert its effects?
d. What prepregnancy advice should this woman have been given?
e. Is it worthwhile ceasing this habit during pregnancy?

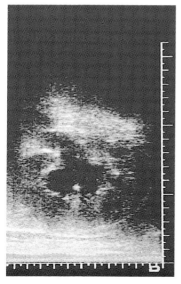

183.

a. What anatomical changes occur in the urinary tract during normal pregnancy?
b. What functional changes occur in the urinary tract?
c. What are the effects of these changes on pregnant women?
d. On which side is a hydroureter likely to be more prominent?

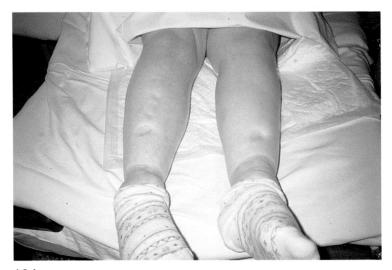

184. **This woman has a blood pressure of 150/110 and ++++ proteinuria.**

a. What obvious sign is evident, and what symptoms may she have?
b. What signs would you specifically look for on examination?
c. What investigations should be performed in this patient?

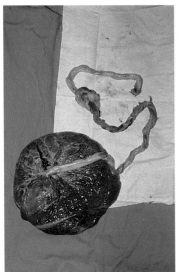

185.

a. What feature is present in the umbilical cord?
b. What are the more common variants of this condition?
c. What are the implications of these different variants?
d. What are the normal constituents of the umbilical cord?
e. What is the significance of the presence of a single umbilical artery?

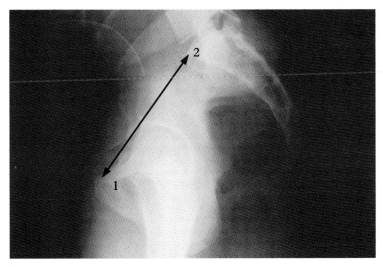

186.

a. What is this X-ray?
b. What are numbers 1 and 2 called?
c. What is this diameter called and what is the normal measurement?
d. What is the presentation of the fetus?

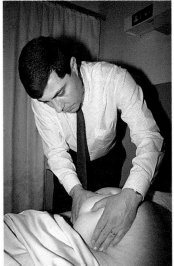

187. What information should be obtained from the 'obstetric palpation' at 36 weeks' gestation?

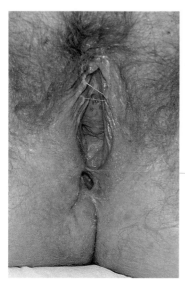

188.

a. What complication has occurred to this episiotomy?
b. What are the predisposing factors?
c. How should this complication be managed?
d. What is the prognosis?

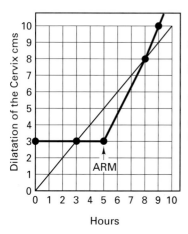

189.

a. Name the phases of the first stage of labour.
b. Which phase is prolonged in this partogram?
c. In what clinical settings may this situation occur?
d. What has been the management?
e. What was the outcome?

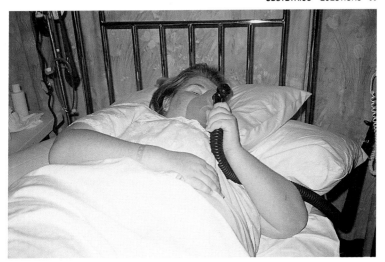

190.

a. What potentially adverse physiological changes can occur secondary to pain in labour?
b. Which form of analgesia best avoids these changes?
c. Which method is this woman using? What are the components?
d. How would you instruct a woman concerning the use of this method of analgesia?

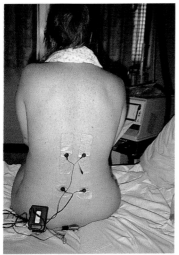

191.

a. What are the causes of pain during the first stage of labour? What are the additional causes of pain during the second stage of labour?
b. Which nerve roots are involved?
c. Which form of analgesia is this woman utilizing?
d. What are the relative merits of this form of analgesia?

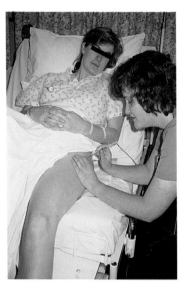

192. This labouring woman is being given an intramuscular injection of pethidine.

a. By what other route may this drug be given?
b. What are the potential maternal side-effects?
c. In what percentage of women will moderate and severe pain, respectively, be relieved?
d. What effects can be seen in the newborn and how are these reversed?

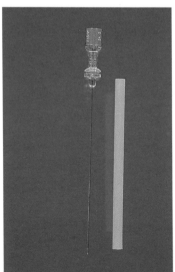

193. This is a 25-gauge needle.

a. For what purpose is it used in labour?
b. What is the anatomy of its insertion?
c. In what situations is it used?
d. What agents may be injected through this needle?
e. How soon is the effect noted?

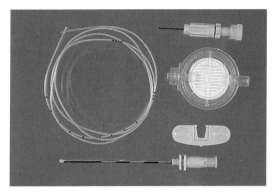

194.

a. For what purpose is this equipment used?
b. Discuss the relevant anatomy.
c. What are the indications for its use?
d. What are the contraindications?
e. What are the complications of its use?

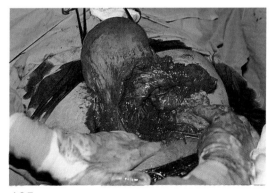

195. This woman is having a caesarean hysterectomy.

a. Would you expect the ovaries to be removed or conserved?
b. What intraoperative complications would you anticipate?
c. If this woman complained of right loin pain postoperatively, what may you suspect?

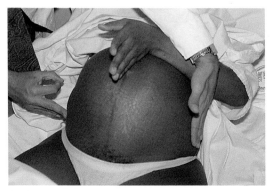

196.

a. What sign is being elicited?
b. What are the other signs of polyhydramnios?
c. What factors are involved in the maintenance of normal amniotic fluid volumes?
d. What are the causes of polyhydramnios?
e. What are the potential complications of polyhydramnios?
f. How would you investigate this patient?

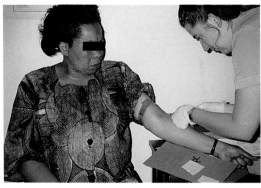

197.

a. What extra antenatal screening test should this pregnant woman have?
b. What conditions will this pick up?
c. What are the thalassaemias?
d. In what populations do the thalassaemias occur?
e. In what populations does sickle cell disease occur?

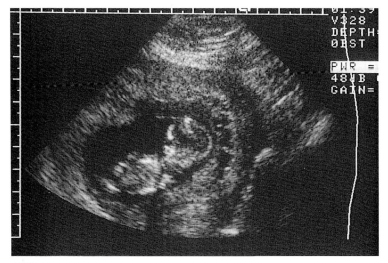

198.

a. How early can an intrauterine pregnancy be detected?
b. When can fetal heart movements first be detected?
c. What is the correlation between crown–rump length and gestational age?
d. What is the usual fetal attitude at this gestation?

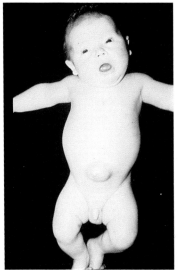

199.

a. What is the diagnosis?
b. What clinical signs are evident?
c. If you are looking after this infant what features might you note?
d. What is the treatment?
e. When do the classic signs usually develop?

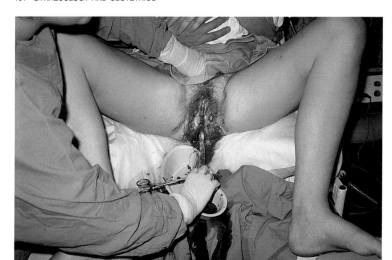

200.

a. What two stages are involved in delivery of the placenta?
b. What are the signs of placental separation?
c. What manoeuvres constitute active management of the third stage?
d. What is the advantage of such management?

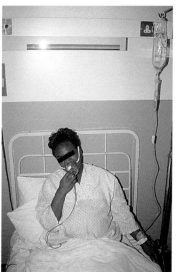

201. This woman is known to have sickle cell disease.

a. What population groups are at risk?
b. What event is she experiencing?
c. What is the antenatal management of a patient with sickle cell disease?
d. What are the principles of management of the situation depicted?

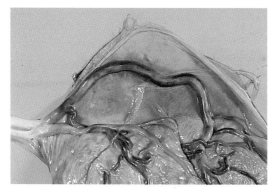

202.

a. What term describes the insertion of these cord vessels?
b. What is a vasa praevia?
c. What are the associated dangers?
d. How would you confirm bleeding of fetal origin?

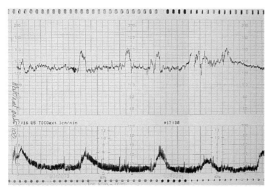

203.

a. Name this investigation.
b. At what paper speed has this been recorded?
c. Which components of the tracing are routinely described?
d. Comment on this trace.
e. What is the overall significance of this trace?

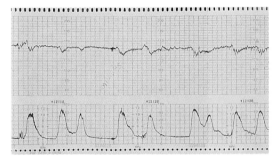

204.

a. How is the fetal heart rate normally controlled?
b. What abnormality is present in this trace?
c. Describe the characteristic features of this pattern.
d. What is the postulated genesis of this pattern?
e. What is the significance of this trace?

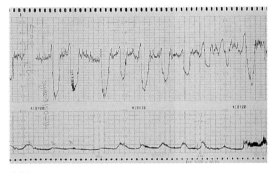

205.

a. What type of decelerations are evident?
b. How would you define this type of deceleration?
c. What is the proposed underlying mechanism?
d. What is the likelihood of the fetal scalp pH measurement being less than 7.25?
e. If this trace occurred immediately after artificial rupture of the membranes, what cause would you want to immediately exclude?

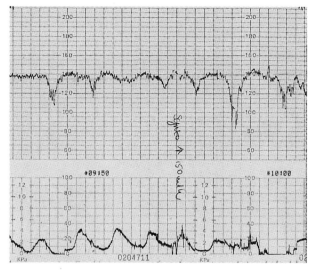

206.

a. What abnormal feature is present in this trace?
b. How is this abnormality defined?
c. What is the proposed mechanism for this abnormality?
d. Would this constitute an indication for fetal blood sampling in labour?
e. What incidence of acidaemia is associated with this trace?

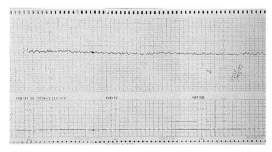

207.

a. What is the normal level of baseline fetal heart variability?
b. Comment on the variability seen in this trace.
c. What are the causes of decreased baseline variability?
d. What is the significance of this trace?

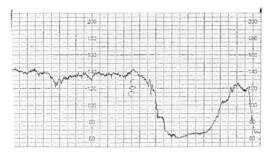

208.

a. Define a prolonged deceleration.
b. What may cause such a deceleration?
c. How would you manage this situation?

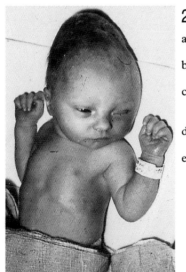

209.

a. What abnormal findings are evident in this newborn infant?
b. How would you define the scalp problem?
c. How is this scalp problem differentiated from caput succedaneum?
d. How may the scalp problem result?
e. What is the natural history? List three potential adverse outcomes associated with this lesion.

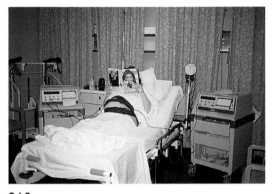

210. This woman with twins is in labour.

a. Which combinations of fetal presentations are commonly seen?
b. How would you manage a twin labour?

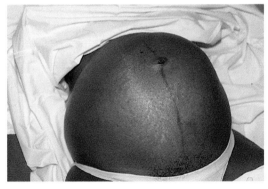

211.

a. What clinical feature is evident on inspection of this gravid abdomen?
b. What is the natural history of this sign?
c. Which population groups are particularly likely to develop this sign?
d. What other common changes are seen in the skin of pregnant women?

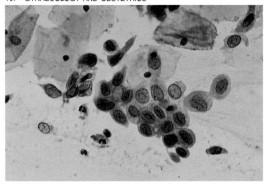

212. This slide shows severe dyskaryosis. The cervical smear was taken from a woman who was 12 weeks pregnant.

a. What is your further management?
b. Is this smear likely to regress to normal without treatment?
c. Is this diagnostic of severe dysplasia?

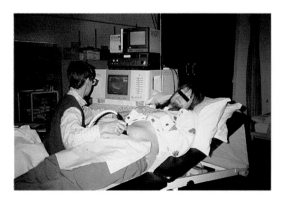

213.

a. What investigation is being performed?
b. In a pregnant woman, what parameter is measured in the first trimester?
c. After 14 weeks what measurements are routinely performed?
d. What must be placed on the maternal abdomen for the correct functioning of the probe?

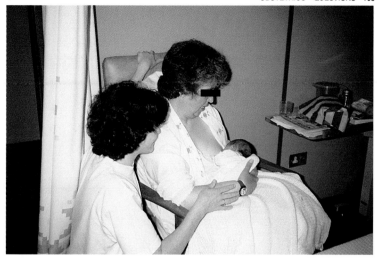

214.

a. What does this slide illustrate?
b. What hormones are involved in milk biosynthesis?
c. How is full lactation in pregnancy prevented?
d. What is the name of the fluid that is produced in the breast in the first few days after delivery? What does this fluid consist of?

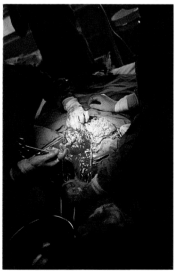

215. This woman is having a caesarean section.

a. What is being removed?
b. What two methods are used at caesarean section to remove this structure?
c. What is the structure to the left of the operator's left hand?
d. What type of anaesthesia has been used?

Answers—Gynaecology

1.
   a. Squamous cells.
   b. Nucleus is enlarged, chromatin is increased and nuclear borders are irregular.

2.
   a. Sims' speculum.
   b. The patient is placed in the left lateral position with the right leg bent and the left leg straight. The upper shoulder is rotated towards the bed.
   c. Uterovaginal prolapse. Cases where it is difficult to visualize the cervix with the Cuscoe's speculum. Suspected fistulae. In gynaecological operations. Antepartum haemorrhage.
   d. Sponge forceps.

3.
   a. Development of the left breast.
   b. Premature thelarche.
   c. This condition is mostly idiopathic, whereby there is unusual sensitivity of the breast tissue to the small amounts of circulating oestrogens.
   d. No treatment is required beyond very careful explanation and reassurance to the parents and child.
   e. Development of breast buds, pubic hair, axillary hair which may not appear until after the onset of menstruation.

4.
   a. VIN (vulval intraepithelial neoplasia).
   b. Vulval biopsy and assessment of the cervix.
   c. Intraoperative bleeding, thermal damage, full-thickness burns.
   d. There is uncertainty concerning the natural history and correct management of VIN. Other options include 5-fluorouracil therapy, wide excision, skinning vulvectomy, simple vulvectomy.
   e. Cooling of the vulva, appropriate analgesia, and Sitz baths. Appropriate follow-up needs to be arranged.

5.
   a. Significant fetal abnormality; danger to the physical or psychological health of the mother or family in the event of pregnancy continuation.
   b. Dilatation and evacuation, suction evacuation (prostaglandins also may be used with these two methods), mifepristone; in the second trimester, intra- or extrauterine prostaglandins and hysterotomy.
   c. Haemorrhage (primary or secondary), uterine perforation,

cervical trauma, intraoperative anaesthetic mishaps. Retained products of conception, venous thromboembolism.
  d. Asherman's syndrome, chronic pelvic inflammatory disease, infertility, cervical incompetence, regret, prolonged grief reaction.

6.
  a. Intrauterine contraceptive devices.
  b. Endometrial sterile inflammatory reaction which inhibits implantation. Sperm migration and ovum transport are altered.
  c. Undiagnosed genital tract bleeding, pregnancy, pelvic infection, major structural abnormalities and Wilson's disease (copper devices).
  d. Aseptic technique, uterus sounded, anterior lip of the cervix is grasped with a volsellum forceps and the device is inserted in the uterine cavity to the predetermined length and the strings are cut.
  e. Immediate complications: pain, vasovagal shock, uterine perforation. Late complications: infection, menorrhagia, expulsion and male dyspareunia (!).
  f. Every 5 years.

7.
  a. Candidal infection (thrush).
  b. Itching and vaginal discharge.
  c. Microbiological swab.
  d. Antifungal agents such as clotrimazole or econazole.
  e. After positively confirming the diagnosis, both partners should be treated concomitantly. The female partner should be treated with a powerful oral agent such as fluconazole.

8.
  a. Rickets.
  b. The bones are poorly mineralized.
  c. Their pelves may be deformed.

9.
  a. Ovarian mass, uterine fibroids, tubo-ovarian abscess, endometrioma, pregnancy.
  b. Full bladder, diverticular abscess, secondary deposits from a primary breast or gastrointestinal (upper or lower) carcinoma.
  c. History: abdominal discomfort, gastrointestinal symptoms, urinary frequency, weight loss, pelvic pressure, abnormal bleeding, backache, dyspareunia, constipation.
     Examination: lymphadenopathy, breasts, pleural effusions, hepatomegaly, ascites, vaginal and rectal examinations.
     Investigations: should be tailored to the particular presentation. May include chest X-ray, abdominal X-ray, upper gastrointestinal endoscopy, ultrasound scan, serum

tumour markers, liver function tests, barium enema. The definitive diagnosis is made at laparotomy.

10.
a. Gram-negative intracellular diplococci.
b. Gonorrhoea.
c. Urethritis, cervicitis which may ascend into the upper genital tract, anorectal and pharyngeal infection. Septic gonococcal arthritis usually involves the knee.
d. Demonstration of the organism in culture.
e. Exclude concomitant infection, appropriate antibiotic therapy, cessation of sex during treatment, tracing of sexual contacts, follow-up for test-of-cure.

11.
a. It is an endeavour to objectively measure the menstrual blood loss.
b. 30–80 ml.
c. This clearly reflects menorrhagia.
d. Most often no cause found. The known causes include fibroids, endometrial polyps, adenomyosis, endometriosis, chronic pelvic inflammatory disease, intrauterine contraceptive devices and endometrial hyperplasia or carcinoma. Endocrine and coagulation disorders are rarely found.
e. Full blood count. Thereafter investigations are determined by the patient's age, and anyone over 35 years of age warrants endometrial sampling. Further investigations such as clotting screen, etc. would be determined by the particular clinical setting. Treatment options are as follows:
  • *Medical*: non-steroidal anti-inflammatory agents, oral contraceptive pill, progestogens, antifibrinolytic agents, danazol.
  • *Surgical*: endometrial ablation/resection, hysterectomy.

12.
a. Female circumcision.
b. Difficulty with micturition, painful menstruation and dyspareunia.
c. Difficulty with cervical assessment and obstructed labour at the outlet.
d. Labioplasty.
e. Anterior episiotomy.

13.
a. Enlargement of the pituitary fossa and double flooring of the fossa.
b. Pituitary adenoma. Secondary amenorrhoea, infertility and galactorrhoea.
c. Serum prolactin, visual fields, and thyroid function tests, CT of the fossa.
d. Drugs (e.g. phenothiazines, metoclopramide, methyldopa),

other pituitary and hypothalamic tumours, primary hypothyroidism, pregnancy.
   e. Bromocriptine, hypophysectomy, and radiation therapy.

14.
a. The vagina.
b. Rhabdomyosarcoma.
c. The first 5 years of life. Peak incidence at around 3 years of age.
d. This usually presents as a grape-like mass which extrudes from the vagina.
e. Extension to the uterus, parametrium and regional nodes.
f. The recent approach has consisted of conservative surgery together with pre- or postoperative chemotherapy and radiation.

15.
a. Cervical smear test. This is a screening test to detect abnormal cervical cells.
b. Aylesbury spatula.
c. Normal recall is 3-yearly.
d. Transformation zone.
e. The smear must be taken quickly, in the absence of blood, smeared (thinly and evenly) across a glass slide and fixed immediately.

16.
a. Vulval carcinoma.
b. Postmenopausal women.
c. Squamous cell carcinoma.
d. Lymphatic spread to the superficial and deep inguinal and femoral nodes and then to the external iliac nodes. Direct spread occurs to vagina, urethra and anus.
e. Radical excision with en bloc dissection of the draining nodes on both sides.

17.
a. Basal Body Temperature chart.
b. There is a small drop in the temperature on day 14, followed by a rise in the temperature of approximately 0.6°C which persists for 12 days. Timing of intercourse appears to have been appropriate.
c. Ovulation.
d. Day 21 progesterone (in a 28-day cycle).

18.
a. Vaginoperineal fistula.
b. Obstetric trauma, either unrecognized or imperfectly repaired.
c. Inclusion of the rectum with a suture during episiotomy repair or perineorrhaphy, Crohn's disease, extension of a pelvic or diverticular abscess, post radiation therapy.

19.
a. Uterine pseudogestational sac, true gestational sac containing a fetus in the right adnexum.
b. Low abdominal pain with vaginal bleeding after amenorrhoea, shoulder tip pain.
c. Unilateral abdominal tenderness, uterine size less than dates, cervical os closed, unilateral adnexal tenderness and cervical excitation, a tender adnexal mass.
d. Serial quantitative beta HCG levels and laparoscopy.

20.
a. Congenital tubal abnormalities, pelvic inflammatory disease, tubal surgery, intrauterine contraceptive devices, previous ectopic pregnancy, and assisted conception techniques.
b. Ampulla, other portions of the tube, ovary, broad ligament, cervix, and abdominal cavity.
c. Tubal abortion, pelvic haematocoele, possible tubal rupture, and rarely an abdominal pregnancy that progresses to term.
d. Other complications of early pregnancy, pelvic inflammatory disease, ovarian cyst accidents, bleeding from the corpus luteum, and appendicitis.

21.
a. Systemic chemotherapy, laparoscopic techniques (salpingostomy or injection of embryotoxic substances), open laparotomy (linear salpingostomy, segmental resection, salpingectomy).
b. The original pathology is probably bilateral. Grief/ bereavement counselling may be required. An early ultrasound scan is required in future pregnancies.
c. Risk is determined by the condition of the contralateral tube. Varies between 10 and 15%.

22.
a. Carcinoma of the cervix and endometrium.
b. External beam radiation therapy, brachytherapy (source close to target), intracavitary.
c. Skin erythema and hair loss, urinary urgency and frequency, nausea and vomiting, abdominal pain, tenesmus, diarrhoea, and bone marrow suppression.
d. Proctitis, rectovaginal fistula, small bowel injury with malabsorption and stricture formation, haemorrhagic cystitis, sterility and vaginal stenosis. Secondary malignancies may occasionally be seen.

23.
a. Endometriosis. This is defined as endometrial tissue in sites other than the uterine cavity.
b. Coelomic metaplasia, retrograde menstruation and subsequent implantation, venous or lymphatic spread.
c. Symptoms are secondary dysmenorrhoea, dyspareunia, chronic pelvic pain and infertility. Signs include pelvic

tenderness, +/– pelvic masses or nodules, and fixed retroversion of the uterus.

d. Biopsy of the lesion.

e. At laparoscopy.

24.

a. The person illustrated has good breast development but no pubic hair.

b. Testicular feminization.

c. The person is a 46,XY individual with androgen insensitivity.

d. Usually after puberty with normal breast development and primary amenorrhoea.

e. Absent or scanty axillary hair, normal vulva, short blind vagina with no cervix. Absent uterus. Testes are found in either the abdomen, the groins, or occasionally in the labia.

25.

a. Surgical specimen showing uterus, tubes and ovaries and an endometrial polyp.

b. No symptoms, abnormal vaginal bleeding, postmenopausal bleeding. If they protrude through the cervix they may cause dysmenorrhoea or postcoital bleeding.

c. May be detected on visual examination. At hysteroscopy they will be seen directly, and at D&C they may be felt with an instrument. An ultrasound scan may also detect them.

d. They may be removed using polyp forceps but ideally they should be removed with an operating hysteroscope.

26.

a. The primary action is to prevent ovulation, and this is supplemented by contraceptive actions at the endometrial and mucus levels and also in the fallopian tube.

b. No. There is a high level initially which declines thereafter.

c. Failure rarely occurs.

d. Highly effective and convenient; diminished incidence of heavy bleeding, anaemia, dysmenorrhoea, premenstrual tension symptoms, endometriosis.

e. Breakthrough bleeding, delay in the return of fertility, weight gain, galactorrhoea and mild androgenic effects.

27.

a. Colposcopy.

b. Abnormal smear, female offspring of women who ingested stilboestrol antenatally, suspicion of vaginal/vulval intraepithelial neoplasia.

c. The cervix is viewed with a bivalve speculum. Acetic acid is applied to the cervix which is then inspected. A colposcopically-directed biopsy is usually taken.

d. The need for the examination should be explained and, if

there is no suspicion of invasive cancer, this should be clearly stated. An explanation of the procedure should be given in nonmedical terms. If the smear result has revealed the presence of wart virus, the sexually transmissible nature of this organism needs to be discussed. The current partner may also need to be checked, and condoms should be worn with any future new partners.

28.
a. Fibroids.
b. Menorrhagia, dysmenorrhoea and distended abdomen.
c. Gonadotrophin-releasing hormone analogues.

29.
a. Clitoral hypertrophy.
b. Atrophy of the breasts and genital tract, male-type baldness, muscular development, hirsutism, and deepening of the voice.
c. Exogenous androgens, late-onset congenital adrenal hyperplasia, androgen-producing tumours of the adrenal cortex or ovary, 5 alpha reductase deficiency and occasionally Cushing's syndrome.
d. Ovary (25%), adrenal gland (25%) and peripheral conversion of testosterone precursors (50%).

30.
a. *History*: onset and duration of symptoms, pubertal and menstrual history, family history and medication intake. *Examination*: weight, blood pressure, signs of virilism, hirsutism or general endocrinopathy, vaginal examination. *Investigations*: serum free testosterone, other appropriate hormone assays as suggested by the history and examination, pelvic (ovarian) ultrasound and, if clinically indicated, computerized tomography scan of adrenal glands, laparoscopy.
b. An androgen-producing tumour of the left ovary.
c. Androblastomas (Sertoli cell and/or Leydig cell tumours), lipoid cell tumours, hilar cell tumours and occasionally metastatic tumours of the ovaries.
d. All signs regress apart from deepening of the voice.

31.
a. Herpes genitalis.
b. Pain, dyspareunia, dysuria, erythema, oedema, vesicles, painful ulcers, inguinal lymphadenopathy.
c. Confirm diagnosis, admit to hospital, analgesia, catheterization if required, salt water baths, topical local anaesthetic, treatment of secondary infection. Acyclovir can help if commenced early. Explanation of the diagnosis and the natural history.
d. If a woman with active herpes presents in labour, delivery

by caesarean section is indicated if the membranes are
intact or have been ruptured for less than 4 hours.

32.
a. Carcinoma of the cervix.
b. The mean age is 52 years. Bimodal distribution with peaks
   at 35–39 years and 60–64 years.
c. Intermenstrual, postcoital or postmenopausal bleeding, and
   abnormal vaginal discharge.
d. Direct invasion into surrounding structures (vagina, uterine
   body, parametrium). Lymphatic and haematogenous
   metastasis.
e. The neck and groin nodes should be checked. Chest X-ray,
   intravenous pyelogram, examination under anaesthetic
   (cystoscopy, bimanual rectovaginal examination, cervical
   biopsy, dilatation and curettage). Additional procedures may
   include a skeletal X-ray and proctoscopy.
f. *Stage 1*: carcinoma confined to the cervix.
   Stage 2: spread to either the upper two-thirds of the vagina
   or the parametrium but without extension to the pelvic side
   wall.
   Stage 3: involvement of the lower third of the vagina,
   extension to the pelvic side wall and all cases with
   hydronephrosis or a nonfunctioning kidney.
   Stage 4: spread to adjacent structures such as bladder or
   rectum or spread to distant organs.

33.
a. Cuscoe's.
b. Dorsal position.
c. The labia are parted with the left hand in order to visualize
   the introitus. The speculum is inserted and rotated
   clockwise with the blades together in a posteroinferior
   direction. Once the speculum is in place the blades are
   separated and the cervix is visualized between the blades.
d. Bimanual examination.

34.
a. Oestrogenic pattern.
b. Superficial cells.
c. High.
d. In women of reproductive age group or women taking
   oestrogens. Women with an oestrogen-producing tumour.

35.
a. An orchidometer.
b. Assessment of testicular volume.
c. The normal testes are equal in size, ovoid, smooth, firm
   and sensitive to even gentle palpation.
d. The mean size of the testis is 4.5 cm in length, and 2.5 cm
   in width. The normal adult testicular volume is greater than
   15 ml.

e. Previous injury or infection, hypogonadal states, irradiation, chemotherapy treatment, previous torsion with vascular damage, old age, chronic liver disease, and myotonic dystrophy.

36.
a. Benign cystic teratoma (dermoid).
b. In young females particularly between the ages of 20 and 30 years.
c. This lesion derives from the primary germ cell layers and can contain structures such as hair, epidermis, cartilage, bone and, of course, teeth. Many other structures can also be found.
d. 10%. The contralateral ovary must always be inspected.
e. Malignant germ cell tumours are rare, especially in young females.

37.
a. A colposcope. It shows a normal cervix.
b. Normal saline, acetic acid, and Lugol's iodine.
c. Abnormal cells. This is a cytological diagnosis.
d. This is a histological term and describes a lesion in which part of the thickness of the epithelium is replaced by cells showing varying degrees of nuclear atypia.

38.
a. Hirsutism.
b. The Ferriman and Gallway system, in which various parts of the body are graded for the degree of hair growth.
c. Idiopathic, ovarian (polycystic ovarian disease, androgen-producing tumours), adrenal (Cushing's syndrome, congenital adrenal hyperplasia, androgen-secreting tumours), drugs.
d. Serum testosterone, LH, FSH, SHBG.
e. Reassurance, local treatment, bleaching agents, plucking, shaving, waxing, electrolysis, drugs (oral contraceptive pill, cyproterone acetate, spironolactone). Drug therapy must be for a minimum period of 18 months.

39.
a. Pessaries.
b. Shelf, Hodge, ring pessary.
c. Shelf, ring pessary: uterovaginal prolapse (patient declines or is unsuitable for surgery); while awaiting surgery or in order to aid healing of decubitus ulceration; in pregnancy. Hodge pessary: this is used in order to antevert a retroverted uterus.
d. Vaginal discharge, ulceration, vaginal bleeding, discomfort, impaction if neglected.
e. 4–6 monthly.

40.
a. Human immunodeficiency virus infection.
b. Homosexual men, intravenous drug abusers, people who have received blood transfusions, partners of the foregoing, and the fetus of an infected mother.
c. Blood, semen, saliva, tears, urine, cervical secretions, amniotic fluid, and breast milk.
d. The ELISA test, and the Western blot.

41.
a. Laparoscopy.
b. Carbon dioxide.
c. Any organs that are within the peritoneal cavity.
d. The bladder must be emptied and an EUA must be performed.

42.
a. CIN 3 and normal squamous epithelium.
b. No.
c. Yearly smears.
d. Severe dyskaryosis.

43.
a. Left fractured neck of femur.
b. Osteoporosis.
c. The spine, radius, neck of femur.
d. Prolonged oestrogen deficiency, steroids, hyperparathyroidism.
e. Significant morbidity and a 20% mortality in the first year.

44.
a. Osteoporosis and vertebral crush fracture.
b. Back pain, loss of height; in some cases no symptoms.
c. Early menopause, white Caucasian, family history, past history of prolonged amenorrhoea or oligomenorrhoea.
d. Trabecular bone.
e. Anxiety about going out of doors and fear of further fractures, depression, difficulty in obtaining clothes to fit and respiratory problems if the rib cage rests on the pelvic brim.

45.
a. Bone densitometry.
b. Mid 30s (although this is somewhat contentious).
c. Adequate calcium intake and weightbearing exercise.
d. Less than 1% per year.
e. 1–6% per year or greater (typically 2–3%).

46.
a. Dual energy X-ray absorptiometry.
b. Bone mass.
c. Single photon absorptiometry, dual photon absorptiometry, quantitative computer tomography, plain X-ray and ultrasound.

    d. Ward's triangle is an area in the neck of femur which measures the earliest site of postmenopausal bone loss.

    e. Decreased scanning time, increased precision.

47.
    a. Insertion of an implant.

    b. Oestradiol or testosterone.

    c. As a form of hormone replacement therapy.

    d. Every 6 months.

    e. If the woman has a uterus she should have 12 days of progestogens each month.

48.
    a. Any combination of distressing physical or psychological symptoms which occur cyclically prior to menstruation and regress or disappear after menstruation.

    b. Symptoms may be physical (breast tenderness, bloating, peripheral oedema, weight gain, headache), affective (irritability, labile mood, anger) cognitive (decreased concentration, indecision), autonomic (nausea, palpitations) and behavioural (poor impulse control, criminal behaviour, social isolation).

    c. Careful history and examination and a prospective daily self-assessment record with an estimation of relative symptom severity for a period of 3 months.

    d. Counselling, dietary modification, stress reduction, medications (pyridoxine, combined oral contraceptive pill, progesterone, bromocriptine, prostaglandin synthetase inhibitors, danazol, Depo-Provera, evening primrose oil, LHRH agonists, spironolactone), bilateral oophorectomy (extreme cases).

49.
    a. Turner's syndrome.

    b. 45, X0.

    c. Short stature, webbed neck, increased carrying angle, sexual infantilism, primary amenorrhoea and widely spaced nipples.

    d. No.

    e. Ultrasound scan (cystic hygroma), chorionic villus sampling, amniocentesis, cordocentesis.

50.
    a. Vaginal septum.

    b. Incomplete fusion of the Müllerian ducts or the synovaginal bulbs do not undergo complete canalization.

    c. Difficulty with insertion of tampons and dyspareunia.

    d. Double cervix and renal tract abnormalities. An IVP or renal ultrasound ought to be performed.

    e. Obstruction of descent in labour. A curiosity is occasionally seen whereby a breech may sit astride a partial septum.

51.
a. Cervical brush.
b. Endocervical canal.
c. When the transformation zone is in the endocervical canal, e.g. postmenopausal women, post cone biopsy. It may also be used in order to obtain an endocervical specimen for chlamydia testing.

52.
a. Hydropic vesicles.
b. Trophoblastic disease.
c. Amenorrhoea followed by vaginal bleeding. Exaggerated symptoms of pregnancy.
d. Typical signs of pregnancy. Uterine size variable but normally larger than dates. Absent fetal heart sounds.
e. Confirm diagnosis with ultrasound scan. Suction evacuation of uterus. Careful monitoring of hCG level. Registration with an appropriate centre. Advise avoidance of pregnancy for a year.

53.
a. Hysteroscopy.
b. CO_2, glycine or normal saline.
c. Visualize the endometrial cavity. Procedures can also be performed through the hysteroscope, for example removal of endometrial polyps or endometrial ablation.

54.
a. Intravenous pyelogram (IVP).
b. Bilateral dilatation of the pelvicalyceal system. The right ureter is easily seen until the pelvic brim. Only the proximal portion of the left ureter can be seen. There is an extrinsic mass effect on the bladder.
c. Urinary urgency, frequency, and symptoms secondary to renal tract infection.
d. Fibroid uterus, ovarian mass.

55.
a. Endometriosis.
b. Ovaries, pouch of Douglas, uterosacral ligaments.
c. Expectant, medical (continuous progesterone therapy, continuous oral contraceptives, danazol, LHRH analogues), surgery (laparoscopic diathermy or laser, open surgery which can range from removal of a simple endometrioma to pelvic clearance).
d. There is a theoretical risk of reactivation of remaining endometriotic deposits, but hormone replacement can be prescribed.

56.
a. Vaginal cyst.
b. Bartholin's cyst, endometrioma, Müllerian duct remnant cysts, Gartner's duct cyst (Wolffian structure). Occasionally this appearance may be mistaken for uterovaginal prolapse.

c. Dyspareunia, difficulty with tampon insertion, sensation of fullness in vagina.

d. Excision of the cyst or marsupialization.

57.
a. Acetic acid.
b. There is a clearly defined area of aceto white.
c. Minor lesion.
d. Nuclear atypia confined to the basal third of the epithelium.
e. Yes.

58.
a. Irregular mass infiltrating the anterior wall of the vagina.
b. Vesico-vaginal fistula.
c. Abnormal connection between the epithelial surfaces of the bladder and the vagina.
d. Post-gynaecological surgery, carcinoma, post radiation therapy, following protracted obstructed labour.
e. Excise the fistulous tract and surrounding abnormal tissue and repair carefully in layers without any tension; continuous drainage of the bladder postoperatively.

59.
a. Squamous cells.
b. Presence of lactobacilli, oestrogen, glycogen, absence of infection.
c. Postmenopausal women (natural or following oophorectomy), prepubertal, post radiation therapy, after the use of hypo-oestrogenic drugs and lactation.

60.
a. Suprapubic bladder drainage.
b. Redivac drain.
c. Previous McBurney's scar and one assumes recent midline incision.
d. The catheter is able to be clamped and when the filling sensation occurs the woman is able to attempt micturition. If she is unsuccessful the catheter can be unclamped. If an intraurethral catheter is used then recatheterization must occur each time.

61.
a. Ultrasound-guided transvaginal (most popular) or transabdominal-trans-vesical oocyte retrieval; laparoscopic retrieval.
b. Controlled ovarian hyperstimulation.
c. Tubal blockage.
d. Male factor infertility (oligospermia), cervical factor, immunological factor, unexplained infertility and continuing infertility after treatment of endometriosis or tubal surgery.

62.
a. 4%.
b. Haematogenous.

c. Lungs, vagina, pelvis, brain, and liver.

d. Full history and examination, quantitative βhCG, liver and renal function tests, full blood count, chest X-ray and pelvic ultrasound or CT scan. Liver scan, CT scan of the head and cerebrospinal fluid hCG level may also be required.

e. Anatomical stage, age, antecedent pregnancy, hCG level, ABO blood group, size, site and number of lesions.

63.
a. Normal.

b. Three days abstinence from ejaculation, rapid transport to the laboratory of a specimen obtained by masturbation.

c. Aspiration of a sample of cervical mucus around the time of ovulation within 6 hours of intercourse.

d. Positive test: motile sperm in cervical mucus. This excludes cervical problem and confirms vaginal intercourse has occurred. A negative test can be caused by many factors other than mucus hostility, for example poor timing or infection.

64.
a. Absence of periods for six months in a previously menstruating woman.

b. Hypothalamus, pituitary, endocrine (thyroid, adrenal), ovary, genital outflow tract.

c. Anorexia nervosa. Hypothalamus.

d. Serum prolactin and FSH levels. Thyroid function test. Further investigations are determined by the clinical features and results of the baseline tests.

65.
a. This is an X-ray of both hands and proximal forearms.

b. Shortening of the fourth metacarpal.

c. 45,XO.

d. Sexual infantilisim, primary amenorrhoea, sterility, webbed neck and cubitus valgus. Low hair line may occur and the chest is shield-shaped with nipples widely spaced.

66.
a. Undescended left testis.

b. Preterm male.

c. The testes are usually left alone and if descent has not occurred by the third year then orchidopexy is performed.

d. Yes.

67.
a. Surgery and radiation therapy.

b. The size and stage of the lesion, together with the age, weight and general medical condition of the woman.

c. The uterus and cervix together with a cuff of vagina, the uterosacral and cardinal ligaments. In addition there is a pelvic node dissection.

d. *Uppermost tape*: external iliac artery.
Lowermost tape: ureter.

68.
a. Carcinoma of the cervix stage I and stage IIa in a woman who is non-obese, usually less than 65 years of age, and otherwise in reasonable health.
b. The common iliac, external and internal iliac, and obturator lymph nodes.
c. *Early*: haemorrhage, infection, fistula, venous thromboembolism.
Late: bladder dysfunction (hypotonia) and lymphocyst formation.
d. Surgery allows conservation of the ovaries and leaves a functional vagina. The treatment is completed 'at one sitting' and the woman knows that the cancer has been 'removed'. There are fewer chronic bladder and bowel disturbances. Radiation therapy can be used in all stages of disease and in the vast majority of patients irrespective of their general medical condition. Ovarian function will not be conserved and the vagina may become stenosed. Long-term bowel and bladder disturbance due to radiation fibrosis can be seen in up to 8% of patients.

69.
a. A spermatozoon.
b. Head, neck and tail.
c. Seminiferous tubules.
d. Follicle stimulating hormone (FSH).
e. Production of testosterone.

70.
a. 4 per 100 woman years.
b. The teat needs to be squeezed, and the sheath unravelled over the erect penis prior to any genital contact. Following ejaculation the still erect penis needs to be withdrawn while holding onto the base of the condom.
c. Provides effective contraception, portable, easy to use, does not require medical supervision and prevents sexually transmitted diseases.
d. Offer postcoital contraception.

71.
a. Gamete intrafallopian transfer (GIFT).
b. Following hyperstimulation of the ovaries, multiple oocytes are retrieved. Some oocytes are mixed with prepared semen and transferred laparoscopically into the fallopian tubes.
c. Unexplained infertility in the presence of normal tubes, cervical factor infertility, unsuccessful standard ovulation induction treatment.
d. Serial ultrasound scanning of the follicles, serial oestradiol measurements.

72.
a. A corpus luteum.
b. Human chorionic gonadotrophin.
c. Twelve weeks' gestation.
d. Progesterone, relaxin and inhibin.
e. Before 7 weeks' gestation.

73.
a. The diathermy loop has been used to perform a large loop excision of the transformation zone.
b. Diagnosis and/or treatment of premalignant conditions of the cervix.
c. Cervical smear test, colposcopy.
d. Cryotherapy, cold coagulation, radical electrocoagulation diathermy, laser vaporization, cone biopsy (cold knife or laser), hysterectomy.
e. Haemorrhage, infection, cervical stenosis. A discharge occurs following the procedure and the patient should be advised to avoid the use of tampons and intercourse for the duration of the discharge.

74.
a. Usually vague, nonspecific symptoms particularly of a gastrointestinal nature. Pressure symptoms such as urinary frequency may be present, together with lower abdominal discomfort and distention.
b. Signs of cachexia, lymphadenopathy, pleural effusions, breast pathology, ascites, omental cake lesion, mass arising from the pelvis (? fixity).
c. Full blood count, biochemical screen, chest X-ray, CA 125 level, ultrasound scan. Other tests sometimes required include barium enema and endoscopy.
d. At laparotomy.
e. Ovarian epithelial cell tumour (most likely malignant).

75.
a. Condylomata acuminata.
b. Human papilloma virus.
c. This is a sexually transmitted disease.
d. Expectant, podophyllin (with great care), cryocautery, electrocautery, excision (rarely), laser ablation, and interferon.
e. The sexually transmissible nature of the condition needs to be discussed. Obvious lesions can be removed but subclinical disease cannot be cured. Recurrences are possible and the partner needs assessment. Condoms should be worn with any new sexual partners. Regular cervical cytology is important.

76.
a. Severe oligospermia.
b. Infection (mumps as an adult or gonococcal infection) or any operations (inguinal herniorrhaphy or orchidopexy),

medication (e.g. antimitotic agents, sulphasalazine, beta blockers) and alcohol intake.
  c. FSH, LH and testosterone levels. Karyotype may be indicated.
  d. Donor insemination or sperm microinjection.

77.
  a. Ovarian carcinoma.
  b. The main method of spread is via the peritoneal cavity. Lymphatic and haematogenous spread also occur.
  c. The omentum is a frequent site of metastatic disease. Omentectomy may reduce subsequent incidence of ascites.
  d. The main prognostic factors are the patient's age together with stage of the tumour and amount of residual disease at completion of laparotomy.

78.
  a. Areas on the anterior lip of the cervix have been stained white with acetic acid. Mosaicism is seen along with abnormal vessels.
  b. CIN 3.
  c. Either a colposcopically directed punch biopsy or loop diathermy.
  d. No.

79.
  a. Milky discharge from both nipples.
  b. Galactorrhoea.
  c. Amenorrhoea or infertility.
  d. Serum prolactin level and if this is raised an X-ray of the pituitary fossa.

80.
  a. In liquid nitrogen.
  b. Basic nonidentifying information, physical characteristics and blood group are noted. Exclude a family history of inherited disorders. Semen analysis. Infection screen (hepatitis B, hepatitis C, HIV, gonorrhoea, syphilis).
  c. Azoospermia, severe oligospermia, paternal hereditary or familial diseases, severe rhesus immunization (use a rhesus-negative donor), failed reversal of vasectomy, impotence, HIV-positive male partner.

81.
  a. CIN 3 and invasive squamous cell carcinoma.
  b. Assuming stage I carcinoma of the cervix, Wertheim's hysterectomy.
  c. Yes.

82.
  a. Primary syphilitic chancre.
  b. *Treponema pallidum.*
  c. The incubation period averages three weeks but may range from 10–90 days.
  d. Demonstration of spirochaetes by dark field microscopy.

e. Confirm the diagnosis and explain the need for compliance and follow-up. Exclude concurrent infections. Parenteral penicillin, abstinence from sex, contact tracing.

83.
a. Vas deferens.
b. Vasectomy.
c. The nature and effect of the operation together with the potential irreversibility and small failure rate.
Postoperatively, the patient must not consider himself sterile until semen analyses confirm azoospermia.
d. Scrotal haematoma, chronic scrotal discomfort, spontaneous reanastomosis of the vas with consequent failure, spermatic granulomas and development of antisperm antibodies.

84.
a. With chronic administration there is an initial stimulatory effect which is followed by down-regulation of pituitary gonadotrophins and induction of a menopause-like state.
b. Nasal spray, subcutaneous injection, depot injections.
c. Fibroids will usually diminish in size by 50%, with the maximal effect seen in 3–4 months. Surgical treatment of fibroids may thus take place more easily.
d. Endometriosis, ovulation-induction regimes, menorrhagia, premenstrual syndrome, and contraception.
e. Amenorrhoea, hot flushes, vaginal dryness, decreased libido, headache and osteoporosis.

85.
a. Endometrial sampling in order to obtain a histological biopsy.
b. Nil.
c. Pregnancy, chronic cervicitis, current or recent pelvic inflammatory disease.
d. Insert vaginal speculum and clean cervix, apply single toothed forceps to the anterior lip of the cervix, sound the uterus, insert the sampler into the uterine cavity, steady the sampler's sheath while rapidly pulling back the piston, withdraw the sampler and express the tissue into an appropriate transport medium.
e. Uterine spasm or cramping, perforation.

86.
a. Filschie sterilization clip.
b. Tubal occlusion.
c. The patient must understand the implications of the procedure. You must discuss the potential irreversibility, the failure rate, the risks and complications of the procedure, and the small risk of a minilaparotomy being required.
d. 2–3 per 1000.

87.
a. Uterine body.
b. Uterosacral ligaments.
c. No, a small amount of free peritoneal fluid is commonly seen.
d. Large bowel.

88.
a. Hysterosalpingogram.
b. Investigation of infertility (uterine anomalies, check tubal patency), check on tubal patency after tubal surgery and occasionally verification of tubal occlusion after a difficult sterilization procedure.
c. Anaphylactic reaction, pelvic pain (tubal spasm), reactivation of pelvic infection.
d. Bicornuate uterus with bilateral free spill of dye.

89.
a. Chronic vulval dystrophy, a generalized pruritic condition, parasitic infection, contact dermatitis, VIN, glycosuria, psychological causes, candidiasis and trichomoniasis.
b. This varies somewhat. One classification is as follows: hypertrophic dystrophy (with and without atypia), atrophic dystrophy (with and without atypia), mixed dystrophy.
c. Vulval biopsy.
d. Hypertrophic dystrophy usually responds to topical corticosteroids. The atrophic dystrophies can be treated with topical testosterone.

90.
a. Laparoscopy with dye instillation.
b. Investigation of infertility, check on tubal patency after tubal surgery.
c. *Laparoscopy*: general anaesthetic but allows full inspection of the pelvic organs and check on tubal patency. Endometriosis and fine peritubal adhesions also seen. *Hysterosalpingography*: outpatient procedure which outlines the uterus and internal tubal structure, but the false negative rate, due to tubal spasm, is higher. No information regarding the peritoneal cavity. The ovaries of the woman receive a dose of irradiation.
d. Normal fimbrial ends with obvious spill of dye.

91.
a. Threatened.
b. Inevitable.
c. Complete (expelled products).
d. Incomplete.
e. Missed.

92.
a. She has an enlarged uterus with a pedunculated fibroid arising from the left lateral fundus.
b. Benign.
c. Total abdominal hysterectomy and bilateral salpingo-oophorectomy.

93.
a. Golf-ball-sized swelling in the left posterolateral vulva. No associated inflammation.
b. Bartholin's cyst.
c. These cysts result from dilatation of the duct rather than of the gland itself.
d. If infection occurs a Bartholin's abscess will result.
e. Marsupialization of the cyst is the simplest treatment.

94.
a. Endometrial carcinoma.
b. Nulliparity, obesity, hypertension, diabetes mellitus, and unopposed oestrogen therapy.
c. Hysteroscopy and endometrial biopsy or formal dilatation and curettage.
d. Adenocarcinoma.
e. Direct spread to adjacent structures, lymphatic and haematogenous spread and spillage of exfoliated cells from the tubes.
f. Total abdominal hysterectomy and bilateral salpingo-oophorectomy, surgical staging +/– adjuvant radiation therapy.

95.
a. Total abdominal hysterectomy.
b. No.
c. Yes, methylene blue.
d. Chromic catgut.

96.
1 = left ovarian fibroma.
2 = uterus.
3 = right fallopian tube.
4 = surgeon's finger.
5 = bladder.
6 = large bowel.

97.
a. There is descent of the cervix with traction to the level of the introitus.
b. There are two towel clips, one Sim's speculum and two volsellum forceps.
c. First degree uterine descent = descent within vagina.
   Second degree uterine descent = descent to the introitus.
   Third degree uterine descent = descent of the uterine body outside the introitus.
d. Rarely congenital weakness. More usually the longterm effects of childbirth, postmenopausal atrophy, chronic elevation of intra-abdominal pressure, e.g. constipation or chronic cough.
e. The patient usually presents with something coming down. Other symptoms include dragging discomfort, a lump which

may be noted, and occasionally bowel and urinary difficulties.

98.
a. Laparoscopy.
b. The operator does not have to bend over; everybody in the theatre can see what is happening; if an assistant holds the camera then the operator has two hands available to do endoscopic surgery.

99.
a. Bacterial vaginosis.
b. A clue cell is evident.
c. The clue cell is an epithelial cell with numerous adherent bacteria. The characteristic organism is *Gardnerella vaginalis*.
d. Thin, grey, homogeneous, odorous discharge.
e. Metronidazole 400 mg orally twice a day for 5 days.

100.
a. Fitz-Hugh–Curtis syndrome.
b. Perihepatitis.
c. *Chlamydia trachomatis.*
d. Signs and symptoms of pelvic infection and infertility.
e. Tetracycline (e.g. doxycycline 100 mg twice daily) for 14 days and ensure partner is treated.

101.
a. Anterior vaginal wall.
b. Bladder.
c. Pelvic pressure, a feeling of something coming down, incomplete bladder emptying. Urinary stress incontinence may be present if there is rotational descent of the bladder neck.
d. Anterior colporrhaphy.
e. Urethral caruncle.

102.
a. Bilateral hydrosalpinges with no spill of dye into the peritoneal cavity.
b. Pelvic inflammatory disease.
c. The terminal aspect of the fallopian tubes.
d. Tubal surgery (laparoscopic or open laparotomy) and in-vitro fertilization.

103.
a. Vaginal hysterectomy.
b. Uterosacral and cardinal ligaments. Other support is provided by the uterus lying at 90° to the vaginal axis and the round and broad ligaments.
c. Bladder, rectum, urethra, ureter and small bowel.
d. Haemorrhage, infection, thromboembolic disease, sequelae of damage to surrounding structures (e.g. fistula), ileus, pelvic haematoma.

104.
a. Fibroid uterus with fibroid arising from the left lateral aspect. The cervix is a separate specimen situated by the ruler.
b. With symptoms of a pelvic mass, namely pain and distention, urinary frequency, or menorrhagia from the fibroid uterus.
c. Probably because the procedure was technically very difficult.
d. Probably conserved.

105.
a. The picture shows a young girl and on her back there are coffee-coloured skin lesions.
b. Cafe au lait spots.
c. Fibrous dysplasia.
d. Albright's syndrome.

106.
a. This is a surgical specimen showing cervix, uterus and both fallopian tubes apparently grossly distended with blood.
b. The patient may have presented with bilateral pelvic pain and perhaps intermenstrual bleeding. Possible pathologies include endometriosis, bilateral ectopic implantation.
c. Yes.
d. Total hysterectomy.

107.
a. Cervical polyp.
b. Postmenopausal bleeding.
c. There is a stroma which contains dilated endocervical crypts. The surface epithelium is usually columnar and mucus-secreting. The surface epithelium may show squamous metaplasia.
d. Polypectomy, hysteroscopy and dilatation and curettage.
e. Twist avulsion as an outpatient procedure.

Answers—Obstetrics

108.
a. Three of the digits have got constriction bands.
b. Amniotic constriction bands occur after premature rupture of the membranes.
c. In this case the distal segments of the fingers appear to have a good blood supply so the prognosis is excellent.

109.
a. Wrong dates, multiple pregnancy, large fetus, uterine fibroids, excessive liquor, adnexal pathology.
b. In the first instance, confirm the dates. Careful history and examination may give clues to the presence of some of the above causes. Investigations would include checking for the presence of gestational diabetes and of antibodies capable of causing isoimmunization. An ultrasound scan would also be required.

110.
a. Leiomyomata. Complications during pregnancy include pain from red degeneration (and this may stimulate preterm labour), increased fundal height, malpresentation and therefore prolapsed cord.
b. Dysfunctional labour, obstructed labour and postpartum haemorrhage.
c. Leave them alone as attempt at removal causes profuse bleeding.

111.
a. Manual removal of the placenta.
b. Informed consent, intravenous access, availability of crossmatched blood, sterile technique and perioperative antibiotics particularly after a long labour.
c. Infection, uterine perforation, retained products of conception.
d. Past history of retained placenta, congenital uterine abnormality, previous uterine surgery (puerperal curettage, myomectomy, caesarean section).

112.
1 = 12 weeks
2 = 16 weeks
3 = 20 weeks
4 = 30 weeks
5 = 36 weeks

113.
a. Increased incidence of congenital malformations, polyhydramnios, preterm labour, macrosomia, intrauterine growth retardation, intrauterine fetal death.

b. Potential worsening of end organ damage, pre-eclampsia, infections, and potential for difficult operative deliveries.

c. Combined medical and obstetric care, excellent blood sugar control (dietary advice and home blood glucose monitoring), early booking with a dating scan, detailed anomaly scan at 18 weeks followed by serial ultrasound scans for growth. Aim for delivery by 40 weeks.

d. Respiratory distress syndrome, birth trauma, hypoglycaemia, hypocalcaemia, and neonatal jaundice.

e. Encourage breast feeding, discuss contraception, stress the importance of excellent blood sugar control being required for three months prior to any subsequent conception.

114.
a. Accessory breast tissue is the most likely diagnosis. This may cause discomfort and embarrassment.

b. Along the 'milk line' which runs from the axillae into the groins.

c. Uncomfortable for a number of days after delivery but then resolves and causes minimal discomfort in about 50% even though lactation continues.

d. Bromocriptine but often excision is required.

115.
a. Twin pregnancy.

b. Approximately 1 in 80.

c. Ovulation induction agents and assisted conception techniques.

d. Hospital care, frequent visits, dating scan, 18-week scan, serial scans for growth. Delivery in a centre with obstetric and neonatal facilities. Iron and folate supplementation.

e. Hyperemesis gravidarum, increased fetal wastage.

116.
a. Episiotomy.

b. This is an incision into the perineum and vagina that enlarges the space at the vaginal outlet and facilitates the birth of the infant.

c. Increased blood loss, perineal soreness, complications such as haematoma, infection or dehiscence, dyspareunia and maternal disappointment.

d. Mediolateral, median, J-shaped.

117.
a. In the presence of appropriate analgesia, the incision is commenced when the head distends the perineum. The incision is made from the midline of the posterior fourchette toward the ischial tuberosity.

b. Skin and subcutaneous tissue, vaginal epithelium, bulbocavernosus muscle and fascia, transverse perineal muscles; occasionally the levator ani muscle.

c. The vaginal epithelium is repaired starting at the apex.

Haemostasis must be obtained and the muscles and fascia are next approximated. Finally the perineal skin margins and subcutaneous tissue are joined. Vaginal and rectal examinations are made and the swab count is verified.

118.
a. Clubfoot or talipes equinovarus.
b. Coexistent abnormalities are common (especially neural tube defects) and clubfoot is a feature of many genetic disorders. Therefore a diligent search for further anomalies must be made.
c. Prolonged oligohydramnios, amniotic band syndrome and abnormal uterine shape or uterine tumours.

119.
a. This is a rapid pregnancy test.
b. Five drops of urine are added to the sample window and the result is available after 5 minutes.
c. The top small square is the control window and a blue line across the centre rectangular window indicates a positive result.
d. For up to 2 hours.
e. The clear view hCG is sensitive to 50 mIU/ml hCG in urine.
f. This test can detect a normal pregnancy on the first day of a missed period.

120.
a. Lower segment caesarean section.
b. Skin, subcutaneous tissue, rectus sheath, parietal peritoneum, uterovesical fold, uterine muscle.
c. Anaesthetic problems, haemorrhage, infection, damage to surrounding structures, paralytic ileus, thromboembolic disease, urinary retention, wound dehiscence.
d. Thromboembolic disease, secondary haemorrhage, incisional hernia, fistulae, uterine rupture in a subsequent labour.

121.
a. The abdominal circumference.
b. At the level of the junction of the umbilical vein and portal sinus.
c. The abdominal circumference helps to determine the adequacy or otherwise of fetal growth. It also contributes to the estimation of fetal weight, and together with the head circumference may help to diagnose microcephaly.
d. The fetal liver, stomach and spine. Further structures in the vicinity include the spleen, pancreas and kidneys.

122.
a. Less than 300 mg per day.
b. Severe pre-eclampsia, renal disease.
c. 0.5 ml per kilogram per hour. Therefore 35 ml per hour.
d. Reduced.

123.
a. Phototherapy.
b. 50%. Haemolysis of superfluous red blood cells; increased enterohepatic circulation of bilirubin before meconium passage; decreased neonatal red blood cell life-span (80 days); hepatic immaturity.
c. Physiological.
   Prehepatic: blood-type incompatibility, infection, morphological red blood cell abnormalities, enclosed haemorrhage (e.g. large cephalhaematoma), red cell enzyme deficiences, polycythaemia.
   Hepatic: drugs, deficiency of glucuronyl transferase, congenital hypothyroidism, hepatitis, galactosaemia.
   Posthepatic: biliary atresia.
d. Development of jaundice within the first 24 hours of life, very rapid increase in intensity, persistence for more than 7 (term) or 14 (preterm) days.

124.
a. Detailed history concentrating on previous pregnancies and their outcomes, and previous transfusions. Blood group, rhesus status and presence of antibodies in the maternal serum are checked.
b. Depending on the antibody level the serum should be retested every month, but if already significantly raised then amniocentesis for bilirubin concentrations or cordocentesis should be performed.
c. Kleihauer test.

125.
a. Grand multipara.
b. Increased incidence of medical disorders with advancing age, malpresentations in labour (therefore a risk of uterine rupture), primary postpartum haemorrhage.
c. Intravenous access, blood for type and screen, extreme care with syntocinon should this be required for induction of labour, continuous fetal heart rate monitoring, prophylactic syntocinon infusion following delivery.
d. Discussion of contraception (including sterilization) is required.

126.
a. Severe varicose veins.
b. Vulva, perianal (haemorrhoids).
c. Progesterone (smooth muscle relaxation), impedence of venous return by gravid uterus.
d. Aches and tiredness of the legs, night cramps, swelling.
e. Thrombophlebitis, haemorrhage.
f. Rest and elevation. Full-length support stockings. Surgical correction, if necessary, should be deferred until after delivery.

127.
a. Partogram.
b. To provide a graphic description of progress in labour.
c. Normal.
d. Primigravida, 1 cm per hour; multipara, 2 cm per hour.
e. Regular uterine contractions, cervical dilatation and descent of the presenting part.

128.
a. Spina bifida results from failure of one or more vertebral arches to fuse.
b. Maternal serum alpha fetoprotein levels and mid-trimester morphology ultrasound.
c. Spina bifida is often a serious congenital abnormality with a range of effects including paralysis and problems with continence.
d. Consume more dietary folate and take a supplement of 0.4 mg folate up to 12 weeks' gestation.

129.
a. The diaphysis only is measured. The femoral head is excluded.
b. The proximal diaphyseal bones, particularly in the lower limbs.
c. After the 14th week of gestation.
d. In early pregnancy, femur length can help to estimate the gestation. Further uses include using the femur length in the biometric assessment of fetuses with suspected intrauterine growth retardation, and in the diagnosis of some congenital limb abnormalities.

130.
a. Obstetric forceps. From top to bottom: Wrigley's, Neville-Barnes', Kielland's forceps.
b. Handle, lock, shank, blades.
c. The lower forcep has a sliding lock compared to a fixed lock and has a cephalic curve only. The middle pair has both a pelvic and cephalic curve.
d. Tilting of the fetal head such that one or other of the parietal bones enters the pelvis first. The sliding lock on the Kielland's forceps will correct this.
e. Traction and/or rotation.

131.
a. Android pelvis.
b. 20%.
c. Heart-shaped pelvis with adequate inlet but reduced midpelvis and outlet measurements. Convergent pelvic side walls and prominent ischial spines. Narrow subpubic angle.
d. Deep transverse arrest is common and if vaginal delivery is achieved, this is often by difficult forceps delivery. Major perineal tears are common.

132.
a. Breast abscess.
b. *Staphylococcus aureus.*
c. Incision and drainage.

133.
a. 14.10 hours.
b. Urine for urinalysis.
c. Yes.
d. The most important function is the detection of proteinuria, but haematuria and glycosuria may also be important to detect.
e. No, because a midstream specimen needs to be collected.

134.
a. Breech presentation.
b. Prematurity, grand multiparity, polyhydramnios, uterine anomaly, fibroids, placenta praevia, multiple pregnancy, congenital fetal abnormality, and intrauterine fetal death.
c. Extended leg, Flexed leg, footling.
d. At term, 2–3%.
e. External cephalic version, assessment for trial for vaginal delivery, elective caesarean section.

135.
a. Cystic hygromas and diffuse hydrops.
b. Cystic hygromas represent an abnormality of the lymphatic system that results in cysts within the soft tissues, especially of the neck.
c. 75%.
d. Turner's syndrome (45, X).
e. The prognosis is poor in the presence of hydrops. Intrauterine fetal death is common.

136.
a. Carpal tunnel syndrome.
b. Pain and paraesthesiae in the distribution of the median nerve.
c. The median nerve is compressed as it passes through the narrow carpal tunnel beneath the flexor retinaculum at the wrist.
d. Hormonally induced fluid retention.
e. Rest and elevation particularly at night and the use of splints can help.

137.
a. Good progress to full dilatation in the first stage of labour. There was a lack of progress thereafter.
b. The fetal head may remain high due to a malposition such as persistent occipito-transverse position.
c. Commencement of oxytocin infusion.
d. Descent of the presenting part and vaginal delivery.
e. Oxytocin should never be given for secondary arrest in a multiparous patient.

138.
a. Gastroschisis.
b. Paraumbilical defect of all layers of the anterior abdominal wall together with evisceration of abdominal organs.
c. The herniated abdominal organs are not contained within a membrane sac and there is a normal umbilical cord insertion.
d. Not associated with other anomalies and fetal karyotype analysis is not indicated.
e. The prognosis is very good and the parents can be counselled accordingly, preferably with paediatric surgical input. Serial ultrasound scans for fetal growth and thickness of bowel wall. The fetus can be delivered vaginally in a centre capable of coping with the neonate.

139.
a. Classical, i.e. upper segment, caesarean section.
b. Fibroid.
c. Three.
d. Caesarean section.

140.
a. Fetal movement chart.
b. From 09.00 a.m. the mother counts each episode of movement and records the time at which the 10th episode is felt. If 10 movements are not felt within a 12-hour period the hospital needs to be notified.
c. Normal.
d. The patient should be invited to hospital for a cardiotocograph.
e. From 16 weeks' gestation in multiparous women, and 20 weeks in nulliparous women.

141.
a. The woman is haemoconcentrated with a raised haemoglobin, raised haematocrit and low platelets.
b. Pre-eclampsia.
c. Delivery.
d. Less than 0.35.

142.
a. Macrosomia.
b. Maternal diabetes mellitus.
c. Dysfunctional labour culminating in shoulder dystocia. The risk of primary postpartum haemorrhage is increased.
d. A carefully conducted trial for vaginal delivery should be undertaken after spontaneous labour with experienced medical staff present at the delivery.

143.
a. Midline defect of the anterior abdominal wall with herniation of intra-abdominal structures into the base of the umbilical cord. The herniated organs are covered by a membrane.

b. Bowel loops, stomach and liver.

c. Associated anomalies are frequently present (cardiac, central nervous system and genitourinary). The incidence of chromosomal abnormalities can range up to 40%.

d. The main determinant of prognosis is the presence and severity of concomitant anomalies. If there are no associated abnormalities the perinatal mortality may be as low as 10%.

e. Associated disorders need to be excluded and the fetal karyotype checked. Vaginal delivery is appropriate.

144.
a. Gestational diabetes.

b. Abnormal glucose tolerance diagnosed for the first time in pregnancy.

c. The hormones of pregnancy induce a level of insulin resistance which increases towards term, and in a normal pregnancy this is countered by a rise in insulin secretion. The tubular reabsorptive capacity is reduced and glycosuria is common.

d. Dietary modification. Blood sugar monitoring. Insulin may occasionally be required. A growth ultrasound scan should be performed at 32 weeks. Aim for vaginal delivery by term.

e. Gestational diabetes is likely to recur in a subsequent pregnancy. In the longer term there is an incidence of non insulin-dependent diabetes.

145.
a. D.

b. A.

c. C.

d. E.

e. B.

f. We refuse to answer this question.

146.
a. *History*: regular painful contractions +/− spontaneous rupture of the membranes.
Examination: descent of the presenting part and progressive dilatation and effacement of the cervix.
Maternal positions for delivery: Semi-recumbent, lithotomy, lateral, knee-elbow or all fours, standing, squatting and sitting.

b. Descent, flexion, internal rotation, delivery of head by extension, restitution, external rotation and delivery of the trunk by lateral flexion.

c. 25–30%.

d. If the cord is loose, it can be slipped over the infant's head. If the cord is tightly around the neck, it can be clamped, cut and unwound.

147.
a. The long axis of the fetus is perpendicular to the long axis of the mother.
b. *Maternal*: grand multiparity, leiomyomata or ovarian cysts, contracted pelvis, uterine abnormality, placenta praevia.
Fetal: prematurity, multiple pregnancy, fetal abnormality, intrauterine fetal death and polyhydramnios.
c. Cord prolapse; if transverse lie is neglected in labour, fetal impaction occurs and this may lead to uterine rupture and maternal death.
d. Admission to hospital for observation. Immediate vaginal examination if rupture of the membranes occurs. Await spontaneous stabilization of the lie or elective caesarean section at 40 weeks.

148.
a. Labour started by artificial means.
b. Adequate indication. Longitudinal lie and preferably cephalic presentation, engaged head, favourable cervix and hopefully fetal maturity.
c. Lie not longitudinal. Cephalopelvic disproportion, major grade of placenta praevia, vasa praevia, cord presentation, carcinoma of the cervix.
d. Failed induction, cord prolapse, inadvertent prematurity, infection, prolonged labour.

149.
a. Precipitate labour.
b. Labour of less than 3 hours' duration.
c. Hypertonic uterine activity or reduced resistance in the lower genital tract.
d. Grand multiparity and extremely preterm labour especially in a multiparous woman.
e. Inadvertent delivery outside hospital, fetal compromise in the presence of strong frequent contractions, maternal and fetal trauma due to very rapid delivery, postpartum haemorrhage.

150.
a. Anencephaly.
b. There is absence of the cerebral hemispheres and cranial vault.
c. Anencephaly can be diagnosed on ultrasound scan from as early as 13 weeks' gestation. The serum alpha fetoprotein levels are raised, and later in pregnancy polyhydramnios is commonly present.
d. The diagnosis is usually made antenatally and termination of pregnancy carried out so that term fetuses with this condition are not commonly seen nowadays.
e. Spina bifida, cleft lip/palate and clubfoot.
f. These infants succumb very soon after birth.

151.
a. Inaccessible lower segment (e.g. lower uterine fibroids or very dense adhesions), nonexistent lower segment, some cases of transverse lie with preterm premature rupture of the membranes, carcinoma of the cervix in pregnancy.
b. Greater intraoperative bleeding, higher incidence of adhesion formation, increased incidence of uterine rupture in subsequent pregnancies or labours.
c. Elective repeat caesarean section.

152.
a. The symphysio–fundal height is measured in centimetres with the tape face down and the 0 end at the predetermined fundus. The tape is run over the gravid abdomen and the measurement is taken at the level of the superior border of the pubic bone.
b. The relationship between the long axis of the fetus and the long axis of the mother.
c. The head is hard, smooth, globular and can be ballotted. The breech is softer, more irregular, less globular and less mobile than the head. It cannot be ballotted.
d. Engagement has occurred when the widest diameter of the presenting part has passed through the pelvic inlet. Abdominally one feels two-fifths or less of the fetal head.
e. Position refers to the relationship of the denominator of the presenting part to the maternal pelvis.

153.
a. Intrauterine growth retardation.
b. Birthweight less than the 10th percentile, head circumference larger than the abdominal circumference, paucity of subcutaneous fat, loose skin, reduced muscle mass of arms, buttocks and thighs.
c. Perinatal asphyxia, meconium aspiration, hypoglycaemia, hypocalcaemia, hypothermia and occasional polycythaemia.
d. Most of these infants survive. Despite the occurrence of some catch-up growth, significant numbers of these children remain small. This phenomenon is more likely with early onset IUGR or when the IUGR has been caused by congenital infection/abnormality or chromosomal anomalies.

154.
a. Fetal scalp electrode.
b. Continuous fetal heart rate monitoring in labour.
c. In the presence of ruptured membranes the distal end of the electrode is brought into contact with the fetal scalp, and the electrical wire contained within it is initially retracted then released by manipulation of the proximal end of the electrode.
d. The electrical signals from the heart are detected directly.

e. Scalp lacerations or infection; inadvertent placement on delicate structures such as the eye in a face presentation.

155.
a. Cord prolapse.
b. Prematurity, abnormal fetus, malpresentation, multiple pregnancy, polyhydramnios, obstetric procedures such as amniotomy with a high fetal head.
c. Feeling the umbilical cord on vaginal examination.
d. If the fetus is alive and known to be normal, immediate delivery is required (caesarean section if cervix not fully dilated). Interim measures include placing the mother in the knee–chest position, maternal oxygen, prevention of cord compression with the examining hand. The question of replacement of the cord which has prolapsed outside the introitus is controversial. Spasm of the umbilical vessels may be caused both by the cold of the air and handling of the cord.

156.
a. Forearm abscess.
b. Intravenous drug abuse.
c. With narcotic abuse, there is an increased incidence of preterm labour and fetal growth retardation. Further complications seen in cocaine abusers include an increased incidence of spontaneous abortion, congenital malformations and placental abruption.
d. Ensure continuity of care, combined obstetric/social work/ dietetic approach, methadone stabilization; with patient's permission, screen for hepatitis B and HIV, serial ultrasounds for growth. Epidural anaesthesia is an appropriate choice for analgesia in labour and the neonate needs careful observation for the development of withdrawal symptoms.

157.
a. Amniocentesis.
b. Ultrasound probe.
c. It allows karyotyping and detection of enzyme defects in the fetus.
d. 1% chance of miscarriage.
e. Chorionic villus sampling.

158.
a. In the first 3 hours in the labour ward there was progress from 3 to 8 cm but in the subsequent 3 hours there was no progress whatsoever.
b. Secondary arrest.
c. Cephalopelvic disproportion, malpresentation or malposition, and obstructive maternal lesions such as fibroids or adnexal masses.

d. Inefficient uterine action.

e. Delivery by caesarean section.

159.
a. This is a transverse scan through the fetal head.

b. The biparietal diameter (BPD).

c. The BPD will predict the gestational age to within +/− 5 days on 95% of occasions in early pregnancy.

d. Isolated choroid plexus cysts appear to be clinically benign. However, serial scanning in order to confirm their resolution is prudent.

160.
a. A congenital diaphragmatic hernia.

b. Mediastinal shift. Presence of abdominal organs in the thoracic cavity.

c. There is a high incidence of associated abnormalities. These include pulmonary hypoplasia, gastrointestinal tract malrotations and chromosomal abnormalities.

d. The prognosis is poor, with a mortality rate reaching up to 75%. The outcome may be better if there are no associated abnormalities.

e. A careful anomaly scan together with fetal karyotyping must be performed. Fetal growth should be followed, and vaginal delivery should occur in a major centre with the appropriate paediatric expertise.

161.
a. Any time from 36 weeks and usually by 40 weeks.

b. Large fetus, abnormally sized fetal head, contracted pelvis, adnexal mass, abnormal uterus, fibroids, placenta praevia.

c. *Clinical observation*: does the fetal head descend on assumption of an upright maternal posture?
Ultrasound scan: fetal morphology, estimated fetal weight, placental location and adnexal masses. Pelvimetry may occasionally be indicated. In the absence of an obvious abnormality, await spontaneous onset of labour and conduct trial for vaginal delivery.

162.
a. Indeterminate, placenta praevia, placental abruption, placental edge bleed, local lesions of the cervix and vagina, vasa praevia, cervical carcinoma.

b. Placental abruption.

c. Vaginal bleeding with abdominal pain. The former may be concealed.

d. Shock, tender irritable uterus with fundus higher than expected for the dates, difficulty feeling the fetal parts, and fetal heart sounds may be irregular or absent.

e. Shock, disseminated intravascular coagulation, intrauterine fetal death or distress, preterm labour, renal failure, postpartum haemorrhage.

f. Admit to hospital and confirm the diagnosis. Estimate the blood loss and severity of abruption. Investigations should include a full blood count, clotting screen and request for crossmatched blood. Intravenous access is required and resuscitation commenced, if necessary. A urinary catheter and central venous pressure line are inserted in most instances. Fetal wellbeing is determined and delivery effected by the most expeditious means. Prophylaxis of postpartum haemorrhage is required.

163.
a. Iron deficiency anaemia.
b. Dietary deficiency in pregnancy.
c. Appropriate iron supplementation.
d. Check for a reticulocyte response.
e. Blood transfusion.

164.
a. Erect lateral pelvimetry.
b. Pelvic diameters and presenting part.
c. Pelvic inlet and pelvic outlet.
d. Breech presentation, after caesarean section for suspected cephalopelvic disproportion.
e. Clinical pelvimetry and computerized tomography pelvimetry.

165.
a. This graph consists of the percentiles related to biparietal diameter (BPD) and abdominal circumference in relationship to the gestation. The graph shows a tailing off of both parameters.
b. Intrauterine growth retardation (IUGR).
c. One definition is birthweight less than the 10th percentile. Symmetrical and asymmetrical growth retardation.
d. Idiopathic.
Maternal: drugs (smoking, alcohol, illicit), systemic disease (hypertension, diabetes, lupus), pre-eclampsia, recurrent antepartum haemorrhages, anaemia and infection.
Fetal: congenital or chromosomal abnormalities, multiple pregnancy.
e. The fetus should be delivered, since there has been no increase in the abdominal circumference between 34 and 36 weeks.

166.
a. Difficult intubation, regurgitation, aspiration of stomach contents.
b. Inadequate fasting, delayed gastric emptying and relaxation of the lower oesophageal sphincter. Gastric emptying is further delayed if opioids have been given. The vocal cords are often oedematous in pregnancy, the increase in body fat

and breast size in pregnancy and the abdominal mass combine to make intubation technically more difficult.

c. H2-receptor-blocking drugs given orally every 6 hours in labour can reduce the acidity of the stomach, and an alkaline mixture is given orally immediately prior to induction of anaesthesia.

167.
a. Pudendal block.
b. To provide perineal anaesthesia.
c. The pudendal nerve derives from S1,2,3,4 and runs in the pudendal canal on the lateral wall of the ischiorectal fossa. A needle passed through the sacrospinous ligament will be in very close proximity to the nerve.
d. Outlet forceps/Ventouse delivery.
e. The pudendal vessels are also in the pudendal canal, and therefore aspiration prior to and during local anaesthetic injection is mandatory.

168.
a. Erb's palsy.
b. Waiter's (or porter's) tip posture.
c. With difficult delivery of the shoulder.
d. Neurapraxia of the brachial plexus (C5, 6).
e. Over 90% recover fully.

169.
a. Systemic lupus erythematosus.
b. Increased early and late pregnancy loss. Hypertension and renal failure, neonatal lupus syndrome.
c. Pregnancy is not thought to affect the longterm prognosis, although pregnancy itself may be associated with more flare-ups, particularly in the puerperium.
d. Appropriate preconception counselling and assessment of disease extent and activity. Drug therapy (may include non-steroidal anti-inflammatory agents, steroids and azathioprine), monitor maternal (blood pressure, renal function) and fetal (growth and fetal heart rate) well being. Optimally timed delivery. Following delivery, watch for maternal flare-up, expert neonatal assessment required; breast feeding may be encouraged depending on maternal drug ingestion, and appropriate contraception should be arranged.

170.
a. Blood.
b. Initial fundal massage. Ergometrine +/− Syntocinon infusion. If ongoing bleeding, examination under anaesthetic. Other measures: intramyometrial syntocinon or prostaglandins. Laparotomy with internal iliac artery ligation or hysterectomy is sometimes required.

c. Transfusion reaction, transmission of infection, and cardiovascular overload.

171.
a. Blood loss $\geq$ 500 ml within 24 hours of delivery.
b. 5% of deliveries.
c. Uterine atony, trauma to the genital tract, retained placenta or retained placental fragments. Other causes include uterine inversion, uterine rupture, and defective coagulation.
d. Initial palpation/massage of uterus. Check completeness of placenta and administration of oxytocin. Resuscitation (venous access, fluid replacement) and blood should be sent for full blood count, clotting studies and cross-matched blood.

172.
a. The placenta remains attached and this could possibly be placenta accreta.
b. Yes, in the presence of an anterior placenta praevia.
c. If the placenta cannot be removed then a caesarean hysterectomy must be performed.

173.
a. Fetal scalp blood sampling.
b. Fetus with a known or suspected blood dyscrasia, amnionitis, situations in which artificial rupture of the membranes is contraindicated. Maternal hepatitis B carriage.
c. Fetal haemorrhage and scalp infection.
d. Fetal capillary blood.
e. pH between 7.25 and 7.35.

174.
a. Forceps delivery. The indications include:
Fetal: fetal distress, forceps to the aftercoming head of a breech, caesarean section.
Maternal: prolonged second stage, maternal distress or medical condition such as heart disease or severe pre-eclampsia, dural tap in labour.
b. Appropriate indication, full dilatation, position known, ruptured membranes, empty bladder, adequate analgesia, no fetal head palpable abdominally.
c. *Maternal*: trauma, infection, bleeding, neurapraxia.
Fetal: trauma, nerve palsies, intracranial haemorrhage.

175.
a. Following delivery there is a fall in the levels of oestrogen and progesterone. High prolactin levels signal the alveolar cells to start producing and secreting milk. Suckling leads to a reflex surge in prolactin secretion, with milk let-down, and oxytocin release. Oxytocin causes contraction of the myoepithelial cells with passage of milk into the lactiferous ducts and sinuses.
b. Water, protein (casein, lactalbumin, lactoferrin,

immunoglobulins), fat, carbohydrates, minerals, trace
elements, vitamins, enzymes and hormones.

c. Cost, convenience, freshness, sterility, correct temperature,
ideal composition, anti-infective properties, portability,
maternal–infant bonding, uterine involution, lactational
amenorrhoea.

176.
a. The midwife is palpating the uterine fundus.
b. A full bladder, and if the patient complained of excessive
bleeding she would consider retained products.
c. She would catheterize the patient and check for urinary
tract infection.

177.
a. Phocomelia.
b. A reduction in size of the proximal parts of the limbs.
c. There is no genetic or hereditary influence; the classic cause
was thalidomide which was used as a sedative.
d. Total absence of limbs.

178.
a. To obtain a fetal blood sample.
b. Needling the fetal heart or intrahepatic umbilical vein and
fetoscopic blood sampling.
c. The fetal karyotype can be determined if this is necessary at
a relatively late stage of pregnancy. Antenatal diagnosis of
haemoglobinopathies, metabolic inherited disorders and
congenital infection is possible. Further indications include
the management of pregnancies affected by
isoimmunization, and fetal blood gas analysis can be
performed in cases of suspected growth retardation.
d. Failed procedure, trauma (maternal and/or fetal), abruption,
infection, intrauterine fetal death, spontaneous rupture of
membranes and preterm labour. Anti-D needs to be given
to rhesus-negative women.

179.
a. From anterior to posterior one can see the frontal suture,
the anterior fontanelle, the two coronal sutures and the
midline sagittal suture.
b. The vertex is an area bordered by the two fontanelles and
the two parietal eminences. The bregma is the large
diamond-shaped anterior fontanelle.
c. The suboccipito-bregmatic diameter of 9.5 cm.
d. The denominator is a defined point of the presenting part
and is used in describing the fetal position. Cephalic,
occiput; breech, sacrum; face, mentum.

180.
a. Meconium staining of the liquor.
b. Intravenous access, blood for type and screen taken,
continuous electronic fetal monitoring (fetal scalp electrode).

Unless the fetal heart rate trace is perfectly reactive, a fetal blood scalp sample should be obtained. If labour proceeds, uterine hyperstimulation and maternal hypotension should be avoided. Difficult vaginal delivery should also be avoided.

c. Paediatrician present at delivery, oral and nasopharygneal suction on the perineum, rapid transfer to paediatrician after delivery for inspection of the cords, and endotracheal aspiration if necessary.

181.
a. A ruptured uterus.
b. Grand multiparity, obstructed labour, oxytocic drugs, and previously scarred uterus.
c. Pain between contractions, vaginal bleeding, maternal tachycardia and hypotension, fetal distress. Contractions may suddenly diminish. If previous caesarean section there may be tenderness over the uterine scar.
d. Maternal resuscitation followed by laparotomy. Specific surgical measures depend on the type, location and extent of the uterine rupture.

182.
a. Smoking.
b. Small baby, preterm labour.
c. Unknown. May be due to nicotine causing vasoconstriction of the placental blood vessel flow, or carbon monoxide binding preferentially to fetal haemoglobin, or it may have a direct toxic effect on the syncytiotrophoblast.
d. Stop smoking prior to pregnancy.
e. Yes.

183.
a. The kidneys increase 1 cm in length, there is dilatation of the collecting systems and ureters, proliferation of Waldeyer's sheath and the urethra may increase in length.
b. Increased renal plasma flow and glomerular filtration rate, decreased tubular reabsorptive capacity although there is increased renal retention of sodium, decreased bladder emptying time.
c. Increased urinary frequency, nocturia, stress incontinence is common, glycosuria, daily protein loss of up to 300 mg can be considered acceptable. Plasma osmolality and levels of urea, creatinine and urate are reduced.
d. On the maternal right side.

184.
a. Gross pitting oedema. Symptoms include swelling, headache, visual disturbances, nausea, epigastric discomfort, vomiting.
b. Confirm the level of hypertension, check the fundi, epigastric/liver tenderness, sacral oedema, hyper-reflexia, clonus, presence of fetal heart.

c. Serum biochemistry (renal function and urate, liver function tests), haematology (full blood count, coagulation screen), 24-hour urine collection (creatinine clearance and protein), ultrasound scan, cardiotocograph.

185.
a. A true double knot of the cord.
b. True single knots of the cord are seen in between 0.1% and 1% of deliveries, while false knots are seen more frequently.
c. False knots do not cause problems, while true knots seldom cause problems because the natural turgor of the cord structures prevents occlusion of the cord vessels. Should a knot tighten, however, asphyxia can result.
d. There is one umbilical vein present with two arteries and Wharton's jelly.
e. There is an increased incidence of fetal malformations and chromosomal abnormalities.

186.
a. Erect lateral pelvimetry.
b. 1 = top of symphysis pubis; 2 = sacral promontory.
c. The obstetric or true conjugate. The normal measurement is greater than 11.5 cm.
d. Cephalic.

187.
a. Inspection (abdominal wall markings, scars), number of fetuses, symphysio–fundal height, the lie, presentation, engagement, fetal position (location of the back), size of fetus, amount of liquor, fetal heart sounds.

188.
a. Breakdown of the episiotomy.
b. Infection, anaemia, nutritional deficiencies, avascular scarred tissue, poor repair technique.
c. Conservative management is best. Sitz baths, antibiotics and normal saline dressings. Resuture of a dehisced episiotomy is very rarely required.
d. The wound usually granulates from within, and in the vast majority of instances heals completely.

189.
a. Latent phase followed by the active phase.
b. The latent phase.
c. Prelabour rupture of the membranes, amniotomy in the presence of an unfavourable cervix.
d. Artificial rupture of the membranes.
e. Normal active phase and second stage followed by vaginal delivery.

190.
a. Hyperventilation, increased oxygen consumption and increased autonomic activity. Increased catecholamine release may impair uterine contractions, blood pressure may

increase, and enhanced lipolysis with release of free fatty acids may contribute to a metabolic acidaemia.

b. Epidural block.

c. Inhalational analgesia with nitrous oxide. Nitrous oxide 50% and oxygen 50%.

d. The mother needs to hold the mask herself, and inhalation of the mixture through deep breaths must be commenced at the very beginning of the contraction. Inhalation can cease once the peak of the contraction has passed.

191.

a. *First stage*: myometrial hypoxia and ischaemia, dilatation of the cervix and lower uterine segment, distention of the uterine body, traction on and stretching of the supporting structures.
Second stage: distention of the vagina, pelvic floor and perineum; pressure on surrounding structures such as the urethra, bladder and rectum.

b. *First stage*: T10–L1.
Second stage: pudendal nerve (S2–4).

c. Transcutaneous nerve stimulation.

d. Nontoxic, easy to apply and frequently effective. The labouring woman controls the level of stimulation and this method of analgesia can be used in combination with other techniques.

192.

a. Intravenous.

b. Nausea, vomiting, sleepiness and feeling out of touch, respiratory depression, hypotension and decreased gastric motility.

c. Moderate pain 70–80%; severe pain 35–60%.

d. Neonatal respiratory depression, decreased Apgar scores, impaired neurobehavioural parameters, and poor feeding. The narcotic effects can be reversed with naloxone.

193.

a. This needle can be used for a spinal block.

b. Skin, subcutaneous tissue, ligamentum flavum, dura mater, subarachnoid space.

c. Instrumental delivery, caesarean section, manual removal of placenta.

d. Local anaesthetic, e.g. bupivacaine.

e. Within 3–5 minutes.

194.

a. Epidural catheterization.

b. The epidural space lies outside the dura mater and contains blood vessels, lymphatics and fat. It is reached via the skin, subcutaneous tissue and ligamentum flavum.

c. Analgesia, operative delivery (caesarean section or vaginal), hypertensive women in labour, maternal heart disease, breech delivery, multiple pregnancy.

d. Patient declines, local sepsis, antepartum haemorrhage or coagulation disorders, allergy to the local anaesthetic agent, active neurological disease, and bony disorders of the lower spine.

e. Dural puncture, maternal hypotension, total spinal block, ineffective analgesia, epidural infection, possibly increased rate of forceps delivery.

195.
a. Conserved.
b. Excessive blood loss, trauma to other intra-abdominal structures.
c. Obstruction of the right ureter.

196.
a. Fluid thrill.
b. Uterus large for dates, difficulty in palpation of fetal parts and hearing the fetal heart.
c. Uteroplacental blood flow, fetal swallowing and micturition.
d. Idiopathic, congenital abnormalities, multiple pregnancy with twin–twin transfusion, diabetes, rhesus isoimmunization, placental chorioangioma.
e. Maternal discomfort, preterm labour, premature rupture of the membranes, placental abruption, malpresentation, cord prolapse, postpartum haemorrhage.
f. Check for the presence of maternal antibodies or diabetes, careful morphology ultrasound scan.

197.
a. She should have haemoglobin electrophoresis.
b. Sickle cell disease and thalassaemia.
c. Autosomal recessively inherited defects in the synthesis of one or more globin chains.
d. Mediterranean and orientals.
e. Negroes.

198.
a. With transabdominal ultrasonography, 6 weeks from last menstrual period. With the use of a vaginal probe, an intrauterine pregnancy can be detected at 5 weeks.
b. Usually by 6 weeks' and certainly by 7 weeks' gestation.
c. There is a very good correlation such that the standard error is +/– 4 days at the 95% confidence limit.
d. The attitude is usually one of flexion but the crown–rump length is taken with the fetus in extension.

199.
a. Cretinism.
b. Enlarged protruding tongue, protruding abdomen with umbilical hernia, lemon skin discolouration.

c. Lethargy, poor feeding, hypotonia, noisy or distressed respiration, hypothermia, and constipation.

d. Thyroxine replacement.

e. Weeks or months after birth.

200.
a. Initial separation of the placenta from the uterine wall and descent into the lower segment is followed by expulsion of the placenta out of the vagina.

b. Show of blood, lengthening of the cord, rise in the height of the uterine fundus; uterus becomes firm and globular.

c. Oxytocin with delivery of the shoulder, clamp and cut umbilical cord after delivery, await signs of separation, the uterus is guarded with a suprapubic hand and controlled cord traction is applied.

d. Diminished blood loss has been documented.

201.
a. Black Africans, Indians, Saudi Arabians and some white Mediterranean groups.

b. Sickle cell crisis in pregnancy.

c. Preconception counselling and test partner. Genetic counselling/prenatal diagnosis for couples where there is a risk of fetal haemoglobinopathy. Full hospital care. Regular blood transfusions to maintain an adequate level of HbA. Maintenance of adequate hydration and prevention of infection are important.

d. Oxygen, adequate analgesia, rehydration, antibiotics, and blood transfusion.

202.
a. Velamentous insertion.

b. Velamentous vessels which lie over the internal os of the cervix in front of the presenting part.

c. The vessels may rupture in labour either spontaneously or after artificial rupture of the membranes. This results in fetal bleeding.

d. Perform an Apt's test, which differentiates fetal and maternal blood.

203.
a. Cardiotocograph.

b. 1 cm per minute.

c. Baseline fetal heart rate, variability, periodic changes and uterine activity.

d. Normal (reactive) trace.

e. In the absence of an acute catastrophe, a reactive trace is associated with a low statistical probability of subsequent fetal demise in the short term following the trace.

204.
a. The fetal heart rate is under autonomic control. The fetal atrial pacemaker is controlled by medullary sympathetic and parasympathetic impulses.
b. Early decelerations.
c. Low amplitude decelerations which are mirror images of the uterine contraction pattern. The nadir of the deceleration occurs at the peak of the contraction.
d. Head compression which results in reflex vagal stimulation.
e. Not associated with fetal hypoxaemia.

205.
a. Variable decelerations.
b. Onset, shape and lag time variable. Shoulders (brief accelerations) commonly seen immediately before and after the deceleration.
c. Cord compression.
d. 15%.
e. Cord prolapse.

206.
a. Late decelerations.
b. The onset of this deceleration is usually late in the contraction cycle, and there is a delay between the peak of the contraction and the nadir of the deceleration.
c. Impaired uterine blood flow with reduced fetal oxygenation and hypoxic depression of the myocardium and central nervous system.
d. Yes.
e. Up to 30%.

207.
a. 5–10 beats per minute.
b. Markedly reduced long-term variability.
c. Hypoxia, drugs (narcotics, tranquillizers, atropine, beta-blockers), prematurity, fetal sleep states, cardiac and CNS abnormalities and arrhythmias.
d. Diminished variability is particularly significant in the presence of another abnormal heart rate feature, in which case the incidence of acidaemia may be up to 40%.

208.
a. Sudden deceleration of at least 15 beats per minute which persists for at least 2 minutes.
b. Prolonged uterine contraction, manipulations (vaginal examination, application of fetal scalp electrode, fetal blood sampling), supine hypotension, epidural insertion or top-up injections, placental abruption and cord prolapse.
c. Place mother on her side, cease oxytocin and give oxygen. Fetal blood sampling may be appropriate if an obvious cause was present and the trace returns to normal. If the trace does not return to normal, delivery needs to be effected.

209.
a. Cephalhaematoma and eyelid palsy.
b. Subperiosteal collection of blood.
c. Caput consists of diffuse swelling of the soft tissues of the scalp whereas a cephalhaematoma does not cross the suture lines.
d. Usually follows traumatic or instrumental delivery but may be seen following spontaneous vaginal delivery.
e. Gradual resorption over 6–12 weeks. Anaemia, jaundice and calcification.

210.
a. Vertex/vertex, vertex/breech, breech/vertex, two breeches.
b. Intravenous line, crossmatch blood, epidural block, concomitant fetal monitoring. An anaesthetist and two paediatricians should be present at the delivery. A Syntocinon infusion should be prepared, and following delivery of the first twin the cord should be securely clamped. A Syntocinon infusion can be commenced in the event of uterine inertia. Otherwise, abdominal palpation is performed in order to confirm a longitudinal lie and with the uterus contracting and a well applied presenting part, the membranes may be ruptured. Only after the second infant is delivered is the third stage oxytocin administered. A prophylactic Syntocinon infusion should be commenced following delivery.

211.
a. Linea nigra.
b. Usually becomes more pronounced during pregnancy and fades thereafter although may not disappear altogether.
c. Dark-skinned people.
d. Hyperpigmentation in other areas (areolae and perineum) and freckles. Facial chloasma, palmar erythema, spider naevi, striae gravidarum, mild hirsutism, and brittle nails.

212.
a. Refer for colposcopy. Providing the colposcopic assessment does not suggest microinvasive or invasive carcinoma, a cervical biopsy would be performed. Further colposcopic assessments would be performed throughout pregnancy and if the appearances did not regress then definitive treatment would be deferred until after delivery.
b. No.
c. No, dysplasia is a histological diagnosis which can only be made after a biopsy has been performed.

213.
a. An ultrasound examination.
b. Crown–rump length.
c. Biparietal diameter, abdominal circumference, femur length.
d. Coupling jelly.

214.
a. A midwife assisting a woman to breast feed.
b. The principal hormone is prolactin. Complete development of the alveolar cells of the breast also requires insulin, cortisol, oestrogen and progesterone.
c. Progesterone interferes with the binding of prolactin to its receptors and the glandular tissue of the breast.
d. Colostrum. The fluid consists of desquamated epithelial cells and a transudate from maternal serum, which has a high content of antibodies.

215.
a. The placenta.
b. Continuous cord traction and manual removal.
c. Omentum.
d. General anaesthesia.

Index

Note: Entries refer to **question and answer numbers**.

Abdominal circumference, 121
Abortion
  spontaneous, 91
  therapeutic, 5
Abscess
  breast, 132
  forearm, 156
Adenoma, pituitary, 13
Albright's syndrome, 105
Amenorrhoea, 64, 79
Amniocentesis, 157
Anaemia, iron deficiency, 163
Anaesthesia/analgesia, 167, 190, 191, 192,
    193, 194
  emergency caesarean section, 166
Android pelvis, 131
Anencephaly, 150

Bacterial vaginosis, 99
Bartholin's cyst, 93
Basal body temperature chart, 17
Biparietal diameter, 159
Bladder
  drainage, suprapubic, 60
  fistula between vagina and, 58
Blood (fetal), sampling, 173, 178
Blood (maternal)
  menstrual loss, 11
  transfusions, 170
Bone mass/density determination, 45, 46
Breast
  abscess, 132
  accessory tissue, 114
  premature development, 3
Breast milk, composition, 175
Breast-feeding, 214
Breech presentation, 134, 164

Caesarean section, 110, 120, 139, 151,
    172, 215
  emergency, 166
  hysterectomy, 172, 195
Cancer, see Malignancy; Premalignancy
Candidiasis, vaginal, 7
Carcinoma, see also Choriocarcinoma
  cervical, 22, 32, 68, 81
  endometrial, 22, 94
  vulval, 16
Cardiotocography, 203, 204, 205, 206,
    207, 208
Carpal tunnel syndrome, 136
Cephalhaematoma, 209
Cephalopelvic disproportion, 164
Cervical brush, 51
Cervix
  colposcopy, 27, 37
  malignancy, 22, 32, 68, 81

polyps, 107
premalignancy (intraepithelial neoplasia),
    42, 57, 78, 81
smear, 15
Chancre, syphilitic, 82
Choriocarcinoma, 62
Chorionic gonadotrophin, human, 72
Circumcision, female, 12
Clitoral hypertrophy, 29
Clubfoot, 118
Colporrhaphy, 101
Colposcopy, 27, 37, 212
Condoms, 70
Condylomata acuminata, 75
Constriction bands, digital, 108
Contraception, 6, 26, 70
Cord, umbilical
  around neck, 146
  blood sampling, 178
  knots, 185
  prolapse, 155
  velamentous vessels, 202
Corpus luteum, 72
Cretinism, 199
Cuscoe's speculum, 33
Cyst
  Bartholin's, 93
  vaginal, 56
Cystic hygroma, 135
Cystic teratoma, benign, 36

Denominator for presentations, 179
Dermoid cyst, 36
Diabetes, 113, 142, 144
Diaphragmatic hernia, 160
Diathermy loop, 73
Drug abuse, 156
Dyskaryosis, 1, 37, 212
Dysplasia, 37, 212

Ectopic pregnancy, 19, 20, 21, 106
Endometriosis, 23, 55, 106
Endometrium
  biopsy, 85
  carcinoma, 22, 94
  polyps, 25
Epidural analgesia, 194
Episiotomy, 116, 117, 188
  breakdown, 187
Erb's palsy, 168

Feminization, testicular, 24
Femoral length measurement, 129
Fertility problems, 61, 63, 76, 79, 88, 90,
    102
Fetus, see specific aspects

Fibroids/leiomyoma, uterine, 28, 54, 84, 92, 104, 110, 139
Fibroma, ovarian, 96
Filschie sterilization clip, 86
Fistula
  recto/perineo-vaginal, 18
  vesico-vaginal, 58
Fitz–Hugh–Curtis syndrome, 100
Fontanelles, cranial, 179
Forceps, obstetric, 130, 174
Fundus, palpation, 176

Galactorrhoea, 79
Gamete intrafallopian transfer, 71
Gastroschisis, 138
Gestational age estimates, 159
GIFT, 71
Glucose tolerance test, 144
Gonadotrophin, human chorionic, 72
Gonadotrophin-RH agonist, 83
Gonorrhoea, 10
Grand multipara, 125
Growth retardation, intrauterine, 153, 165

Haematology
  iron deficiency anaemia, 163
  pre-eclampsia, 141
Haemoglobinopathy, 197, 201
Haemorrhage
  antepartum, 162
  postpartum, 171
Head, fetal, engagement, 161
Heart (fetal)
  rate
    decelerations, 204, 205, 206, 208
    monitoring, 154, 203, 204, 205, 206, 207, 208
    variations, 207
  sounds, 145
Hernia, diaphragmatic, 160
Herpes genitalis, 31
Hirsutism, 38
HIV, 40
Hormone replacement therapy, 47
HPV, 75
Human chorionic gonadotrophin, 72
Human immunodeficiency virus, 40
Human papilloma virus, 75
Hydramnios, 196
Hydrops, fetal, 135
Hygromas, cystic, 135
Hypertension, 184
Hysterectomy, 67, 68, 81, 92, 95, 103
  caesarean, 172, 195
  vaginal, 103
  Wertheim's, 67, 68, 81
Hysterosalpingogram, 88, 102
Hysteroscopy, 53

In vitro fertilization, 61
Infertility, 61, 63, 76, 79, 88, 90, 102

Inflammatory disease, pelvic, 102
Intrauterine contraceptive device, 6
Intrauterine growth retardation, 153, 165
Iron deficiency anaemia, 163
IUCD, 6

Jaundice, neonatal, 123

Kidney
  disease, 122
  pregnancy-related changes, 183

Labour
  first stage, 189, 190
  induction, 148
  pain, see Pain
  precipitate, 149
  second stage, 190
  secondary arrest, 158
  third stage, 200
  twin, 210
Lactation, 175
Laparoscopy, 41, 90, 98
Large-for-dates, 109
Leiomyoma (fibroids), uterine, 28, 54, 84, 92, 104, 110, 139
Linea nigra, 211
Lupus erythematosus, systemic, 169

Macrosomia, 142
Malignancy/cancer, 1, 40, 62, see also specific tissue/histological types and Premalignancy
  cervical, 22, 32, 68
  endometrial, 22, 94
  ovarian, 77
  vaginal, 14
  vulval, 16
Meconium staining, 180
Medroxyprogesterone acetate, depot, 26
Menstrual abnormalities, 11, 64, 79
Movements, fetal, 140
Multipara, grand, 125

Nipples, accessory, 114
Nitrous oxide, 190

Oestrogen
  therapy, 47
  tumour producing, 34
Oligospermia, 76
Omphalocoele, 143
Oocyte retrieval, 61
Orchidometry, 35
Osteomalacia, juvenile, 8
Osteoporosis, 43, 44
Ovarian mass/tumour, 54, 74, 77, 96
Oxytocin infusion, 137

Pain, labour/delivery, 109
  relief, see Anaesthesia/analgesia

Palpation, obstetric, 176, 187
Papilloma virus, human, 75
Partogram, 127
Pelvic inflammatory disease, 102
Pelvimetry, 164, 186
Pelvis
  android, 131
  mass, 9
Perihepatitis, 102
Perineum
  analgesia, 167
  fistula involving, 18
Pes (talipes) equinovarus, 119
Pessaries, 39
Pethidine, 193
Phocomelia, 177
Phototherapy, 123
Pituitary adenoma, 13
Placenta
  accreta, 172
  delivery, 200
  manual removal, 111, 215
Polyhydramnios, 196
Polyps
  cervical, 107
  endometrial, 25
Postcoital test, 63
Precocious puberty, 105
Pre-eclampsia, 122, 141
Pregnancy test/detection, 119
  intrauterine, 198
Premalignancy, 4, 42, 57, 73, 78, 81
Premature thelarche, 3
Premenstrual syndrome, 48
Prolapse (descent)
  cord, 155
  uterus, 97
Puberty, precocious, 105
Pudendal block, 167
Pyelography, 54

Radiotherapy, 22, 67
Rectovaginal fistula, 18
Renal medicine, see Kidney
Rhabdomyosarcoma, 14
Rhesus isoimmunization, 124
Rickets, 8
Ruptured uterus, 181

Salpingectomy, 21
Salpingo-oophorectomy, 92
Sarcoma, Kaposi's, 49
Sarcoma botryoides, 14
Scalp, fetal
  electrodes, 154
  problems, 209
Semen
  analysis, 63, 76
  donated, 80
Sickle cell disease, 197, 201
Sim's speculum, 2
Smoking, 182

Sperm(atozoon), 69
  count, 63, 76
    low, 76
  motility test, 63, 76
Spina bifida, 128
Spinal block, 193
Sterilization
  female, 86
  male, 83
Sutures, cranial, 179
Symphysio–fundal height, 152
Syphilis, 82
Systemic lupus erythematosus, 169

Talipes equinovarus, 119
Temperature, basal body, 17
TENS, 191
Teratoma, benign cystic, 36
Termination of pregnancy, 5
Testicles
  maldescent, 66
  size measurement, 35
Testicular feminization, 24
Testosterone, therapy, 47
Thalassaemia, 197
Thelarche, premature, 3
Thrush, 7
Transcutaneous nerve stimulation, 191
Transverse lie, 147
Trophoblastic disease, 52
Tumours (and undefined masses), 1, 36,
    40, 62, see also specific tissue/histological
    types
  cervical, 22, 32, 68
  endometrial, 22, 94
  malignant, see Malignancy
  oestrogen-producing, 34
  ovarian, 54, 74, 77, 97
  pelvic, 9
  pituitary, 13
  uterine, 28, 54, 84, 92, 104
  vaginal, 14
  vulval, 16
Turner's syndrome, 49, 65, 135
Twins, 115, 210

Ultrasound, 198, 213
Urinalysis, 122, 133
Urinary tract, pregnancy-related changes,
    183
Uterus, see also entries under Intrauterine
  atony, 170
  descent, 97
  rupture, 181
  tumours, 28, 54, 84, 92, 101, 104, 139

Vagina, see also Colposcopy
  bulging wall, 101
  candidiasis, 7
  cyst, 56
  fistulae involving, see Fistula
  hysterectomy via, 103